SUCCESSFUL CHANGE MANAGEMENT IN HEALTH CARE

Change is frequent in healthcare, yet change management is often far from perfect. This book considers the complexity of change within large organisations, explores existing models of change and emphasises the vital role of emotional and cognitive readiness in successful change management.

Despite the plethora of organisational change management approaches used in healthcare, the success rate of change in organisations can be as low as 30%. New thinking about change management is required to improve success in service development, improvement and innovation. Arguing that emotional and cognitive readiness for change requires engagement with the people involved, and a thorough understanding of areas of friction and potential challenge, this book also delves into the neglected issue of emotion, examining emotional labour and emotion and change. It investigates how human emotion can be incorporated into Change Management Models, alongside and intertwined with cognitive approaches, to support effective change. Using the NHS as a central case study, this book incorporates examples of actual change from a range of healthcare settings from acute to primary care, enabling readers to see how Change Management Models can be adapted and utilised in practice.

This is an essential read for students, as future change leaders, and practitioners and managers leading and managing change in healthcare.

Annette Chowthi-Williams was a senior manager in the NHS and is Senior Lecturer at the University of West London, UK.

Geraldine Davis was a senior lecturer at the University of Essex and then Principal Lecturer at Anglia Ruskin University, UK, until her retirement in 2018.

SUCCESSFUL CHANGE MANAGEMENT IN HEALTH CARE

Being Emotionally and Cognitively Ready

Annette Chowthi-Williams and
Geraldine Davis

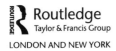
LONDON AND NEW YORK

Cover image: © Getty Images

First published 2022
by Routledge
2 Park Square, Milton Park, Abingdon, Oxon OX14 4RN

and by Routledge
605 Third Avenue, New York, NY 10158

Routledge is an imprint of the Taylor & Francis Group, an informa business

© 2022 **Annette Chowthi-Williams and Geraldine Davis**

The right of **Annette Chowthi-Williams and Geraldine Davis** to be identified as authors of this work has been asserted by them in accordance with sections 77 and 78 of the Copyright, Designs and Patents Act 1988.

All rights reserved. No part of this book may be reprinted or reproduced or utilised in any form or by any electronic, mechanical, or other means, now known or hereafter invented, including photocopying and recording, or in any information storage or retrieval system, without permission in writing from the publishers.

Trademark notice: Product or corporate names may be trademarks or registered trademarks, and are used only for identification and explanation without intent to infringe.

British Library Cataloguing-in-Publication Data
A catalogue record for this book is available from the British Library

Library of Congress Cataloging-in-Publication Data
A catalog record for this book has been requested

ISBN: 978-0-367-65215-9 (hbk)
ISBN: 978-0-367-65213-5 (pbk)
ISBN: 978-1-003-12839-7 (ebk)

DOI: 10.4324/9781003128397

Typeset in Bembo
by Apex CoVantage, LLC

CONTENTS

List of figures vi
List of tables vii
List of boxes viii

1 Change and health care 1

2 Complexity and change management 21

3 A critique of change management theories and approaches 42

4 Critique of change management approaches: behavioural and emotionally centred models 65

5 Emotional labour and emotion and change 77

6 Emotional and cognitive readiness for change 91

7 Emotional and cognitive readiness for change: new thinking 109

8 Applying the AC-W Change Management Model: assessing emotional and cognitive readiness for change 129

9 Planning and implementing service development, improvement and innovation 151

10 Conclusions 178

Index 192

FIGURES

7.1 Diagram of the AC-W Change Management Model 110
9.1 Driving and sustaining forces for implementation of the App 156

TABLES

1.1	Examples of UK Health Policies over the period 1983–1997	3
1.2	Examples of UK Health Policies over the period 1997–2009	4
1.3	Examples of UK Health Policies over the period 2010–2016	5
6.1	Tool for the retrospective assessment of emotional and cognitive readiness for change	101
6.2	Tool for the real time assessment of cognitive and emotional readiness for change	102
6.3	Tool for the prospective assessment of emotional and cognitive readiness for change	104
7.1	Best practice for effective leadership in organisations at all levels, across all professionals, administrative, technical, clinical, managers and executives	117
7.2	Best practice for effective engagement and involvement of people, empowerment, vision building and valuing everyone equally	119
7.3	Best practice for creating inter-organisational communication forums	121
7.4	Best practice for creating a culture of readiness for continuous change	122
7.5	Best practice for affirming and embedding the direction of change in the frontline	123
7.6	Best practice for using a Change Management Model that best fits the organisation's business for change leaders	124
8.1	Participants in retrospective change case study	133
8.2	Participants in real time change case study	135
8.3	Participants in prospective change case study	144
9.1	Assessment of emotional and cognitive readiness for change using AC-W Change Management Model: a summary of readiness for change for Case study 1	155
9.2	Assessing emotional and cognitive readiness for change: a summary of readiness for change for Case study 2	163
9.3	Assessment of emotional and cognitive readiness for change: a summary of readiness for change for Case study 3	172

BOXES

8.1	Case study 1	132
8.2	Case study 2	133
8.3	Case study 3	146
9.1	Implementation of an App to aid patients in primary care to self-manage their type 2 diabetes (a prospective change) – summary of the change process	153
9.2	Redesign of the medical unit to create a medical division (a retrospective change) – summary of the change process	160
9.3	Introduction of a new scheme to attract and retain staff across mental health services (a real time change) – summary of the change process	170

1
CHANGE AND HEALTH CARE

Introduction

This book argues for new thinking on change management in health care to improve its success. Continuous change is now a common feature in health and social care organisations across the globe and the National Health Service (NHS) in the UK is no different. With continuous NHS policy changes of successive UK governments and the enormous resources given to supporting service improvement, innovation and development, the evidence for improved quality, care, productivity and a happy workforce should be obvious. Rather, the evidence points in the opposite direction. The case for a shift in direction for change management could not be more urgent. We explore the failure of current change management in healthcare and how our new thinking about emotional and cognitive readiness for change could provide the energy, motivation and engagement for successful change management. We argue that the incessant policy initiatives are impacting the health and wellbeing of the workforce, the financial health and productivity of the NHS and failing to improve the nations' health. Innovation, service development and improvement are key to improving quality health care and the nations' health but change must be effective to be sustained.

We suggest that successful change management in healthcare is reliant on change leaders addressing the inhibitors to change management and reorientating its focus and energy on people. People are the NHS's greatest resource and strength, and current conditions do not lend themselves to ensuring employee's emotional and cognitive readiness for change. Leaders should consider change and complexities in the NHS and the level of effectiveness of current change management approaches. With the impact of emotional labour on the workforce already high, change is an added emotional burden. The critical role of emotion and change needs to be recognised, acknowledged and addressed. With change having a negative impact on staff, change leaders need to understand the significance of and actively assess for emotional and cognitive readiness for change prior to any change initiatives. Thus, the voices of the workforce will contribute to the preparedness plan for change and subsequent implementation thereby ensuring a smooth transition with staff feeling that they are valued, engaged in the change process and their feelings, views and opinions respected. We outline these ideas in this chapter and explore these in more depth in this book.

In the early part of this chapter, we set out examples of the enormity of policy change in the UK. We introduce some of the issues related to devolution of health care. We include examples of the outcomes and impact of these changes on the health of the nation, on the health and wellbeing of the workforce and on the financial health of the NHS, productivity and lack of sustainable improvement, to provide a background to why people might be suspicious of yet more change and reluctant to embrace change without question.

We continue in this chapter to outline the case for new thinking on how change management could potentially be successful in the NHS. In Chapter 2, we examine change and complexity. In Chapters 3 and 4, we critique some of the many change management approaches, models, theories and tools used in change management. Emotional labour and the key role of emotion and change is examined in Chapter 5. Emotional and cognitive readiness for change, which is potentially the key to successful change management, is explored in Chapter 6, where we introduce the AC-W Change Management Model. We explore the underpinning philosophy of this model and its role in ensuring emotional and cognitive readiness for change in Chapter 7, and in Chapters 8 and 9, we illustrate the AC-W model in practice. The final chapter summarises our thinking on the failure of change management in healthcare and how our new thinking could potentially lead to successful change management.

Policy and the NHS

As an illustration of just how incessant policy change has been, we highlight some of these changes in Tables 1.1–1.3. Table 1.1 demonstrates a selection of the changes to the health service from 1983 to 1997. Some of these were about changes in structure and the nature of provider and commissioner (e.g. Working for Patients, 1989; Health Authorities Act, 1995). Others focused on specific improvements in health (e.g. Health of the Nation, 1992).

The Tony Blair government reforms to the NHS extended to three areas: targets and performance management, inspection and regulation and competition and choice. There have been many criticisms of these changes with their emphasis on these areas as a means to improve health care. Considering the resources, the benefits are mixed. In the area of targets and performance there were stated improvements. There were reductions in waiting times, in health care-acquired infections, and improvements in cancer and cardiac care. While these achievements are positive, there were concerns 'of gaming and, in some cases, misreporting of

TABLE 1.1 Examples of UK Health Policies over the period 1983–1997

Date	Policy/Report	Summary
1983	The Griffiths Report	Consensus management through committee was replaced by general management structure.
1989	Caring for People	Leadership of community care was given to local authorities following the 1988 paper Community Care: an agenda for action and the Audit Commission report making a reality of community care.
1989	Working for Patients	A split occurred between purchasers and providers of health. Self-governing hospital trusts and fundholding GP practices were introduced.
1992	Health of the Nation	Targets were set to improve health in five areas: coronary heart disease and stroke; cancer; accidents; mental illness; and HIV/AIDs and sexual health.
1995	Health Authorities Act	This act abolished Regional Health Authorities and replaced them with NHS Executive offices. District Health Authorities and Family Health Service Authorities were merged.

data to avoid penalties and sanctions under the performance management regime' (Ham, 2015, p. 10). With regard to inspection and regulation, it could be argued that despite regulators visiting the Stoke Mandeville Hospital, Maidstone and Tunbridge Wells NHS Trust and Mid Staffordshire NHS Foundation Trust, there were serious failings in patient care. The benefit of all this change was not seen. The introduction of competition and choice did not fare much better. The question remained: what was the benefit?

Between 1997 and 2009, there was considerable emphasis on primary care and community and integrating care or on introducing specific targets as shown in Table 1.2. Year 1998–1999 saw two other significant changes, the establishment of NICE (National Institute for Clinical Excellence, now National Institute for Health and Care Excellence) and the devolution of health care to the four nations of the UK. Since that time, policy frameworks in England, serving some 84.2% of the UK population (based on ONS data), have differed from those in the other three countries of the UK, creating four systems with different structures, of which NHS England appears the most complex (Dayan & Edwards, 2017). We discuss some of these differences in Chapter 2. Later policies in this period emphasised quality of care, changes in pay and contracts and increased metrics, for example aiming to measure performance through targets and results.

Since 2010, the policy initiatives have continued their relentless pace, as shown in Table 1.3. Alongside policies aiming to promote joint working between services, improve access to care, and promote seven days a week services, are others aiming for significant savings. There are also two very dominant elements during this time. The first of these is the Health and Social Care Act of 2012, which aimed

4 Change and health care

TABLE 1.2 Examples of UK Health Policies over the period 1997–2009

Date	Policy/Report	Summary
1997	The New NHS: Modern, Dependable	A shift of focus occurred to primary care. Clinical governance was introduced. Finance was linked to reform.
1998	Health Action Zones	Early attempts to integrate health and social care. Some 10 areas implemented strategies locally aimed to improve health.
1998	A First Class Service	NICE and CHI (later led to Healthcare Commission and CQC) established.
1999	Devolution	Health systems were devolved to the four UK countries: England, Scotland, Wales and Northern Ireland.
1999	The NHS Plan	Many targets introduced, reforms for improvement of services.
1999	Introduction of Primary Care Groups	Direct management of community services such as health visiting, local payment for services.
2000	Health Act	Joint working between health and social care supported.
2001	Shifting the Balance of Power	This focused on structural change to implement the NHS Plan. PCTs and SHAs were created. The NHS Executive became part of the DoH.
2001	Health and Social Care Act	Aimed to improve performance within the NHS. Changes were made to: regulation of health professionals; pharmacy and prescribing; payments for users of social services; funding of long-term care; CHCs, planning for these to be abolished.
2001	Delivering the NHS Plan	Shift to the notion of a regulated system. Foundation Trusts initiated, provision of services from a range of providers developed.
2002	Care Trusts	Aimed to promote integration of health and social care by introducing commission and provider-based Care Trusts.
2003	New Consultant Contract	Aimed to recognise both flexible working patterns and non-clinical and on call work by consultants, effectively increasing earnings and pensions.
2003	New GP Contract	A new GMS contract linked to Quality Outcomes Framework aimed to incentivise preventative care.
2003	Payment by Results	Aimed to increase choice. Commissioners more able to manage and influence provider activity.
2004	NHS Improvement Plan	18 week target from referral to treatment proposed, and 48 hour GP access target.
2004	Agenda for Change	Introduced streamlining of pay scales across the NHS.
2005	Commissioning a Patient Led NHS	PCTs to lose provider responsibilities (implemented 2009). SHAs reconfigured.

Date	Policy/Report	Summary
2006	Our Health, Our Care, Our Say	Aimed to improve support for long-term conditions, and improve choice in primary and community care.
2008	High Quality Care for All (Next Stage Review)	Aimed to improve quality and safety through quality improvement staff initiatives. Integrated care pilots introduced, with new priorities identified for primary care access.
2009	Personal Health Budgets: First Steps	Aimed to pilot personal health budgets.

to devolve decision making and enable general practitioners (GPs) to take the role of commissioners, with greater choice and competition. The King's Fund report (Ham et al., 2015) describes how from 2010, during the first half of the coalition government, work progressed to enact this policy, but then for the second part, to 2015, the work focused on putting things right following policy failure. Things had to change to reduce the focus on competition, to improve the quality and regulation of care and to put patients and their safety first. The act increased marketisation in the NHS and led to re-organisation, with more hierarchy, greater complexity and confusion amongst staff and patients as to how things worked. Ham et al. (2015) noted the lack of effective leadership.

TABLE 1.3 Examples of UK Health Policies over the period 2010–2016

Date	Policy/Report	Summary
2010	Equity and Excellence: Liberating the NHS	Paved the way for the Health and Social Care Act of 2012 (implemented in 2013).
2010 and subsequently	Quality, Innovation, Productivity and Prevention. The Nicholson Challenge	Aimed for £20 billion in savings within the NHS.
2011	Commissioning Clusters	Aimed to oversee the transition between PCTs and CCGs.
2012	The Health and Social Care Act	Abolished PCTs and SHAs. Created the CCGs and NHS England and established Public Health England.
2013	Francis Inquiry Report	Report into Mid Staffordshire culture and values, established that quality and safety should be paramount, not financial responsibilities.
2013	Prime Minister's Challenge Fund	Aimed to develop models for improved access to GPs through innovation funding.

(Continued)

TABLE 1.3 (Continued)

Date	Policy/Report	Summary
2013	Better Care Fund (Integration Transformation Fund)	Aimed to move funding for social care to local authorities, to support hospital discharge and reduce hospital admission.
2013	Every Day Counts	Introduced standards for seven days a week hospital services.
2014	Five Year Forward View	Population health, quality of care and cost-control described as the 'triple aim', re-emphasis on prevention, aimed for better integration between physical and mental health, between primary and other health services and between health and social care.
2014	Parity of Esteem	Aimed for parity between funding and esteem for mental and physical health.
2015	New Deal for General Practice	Planned for seven days a week GP service by addressing workforce and other challenges.
2015	NHS Improvement	Aimed to simplify the regulatory system.
2015	Sustainability and Transformation Fund	Additional funding identified to support changes in the Five Year Forward View.
2016	Sustainability and Transformation Partnerships (STPs)	Aimed for joint planning of health of local populations through NHS Trusts, commissioners and local authorities working together.

The second element of particular note is the Francis Inquiry Report (2013) into failings at Mid Staffordshire NHS Foundation Trust between 2005 and 2009. This report, although based on one Trust, applies to all Trusts. Standards of care were found to be appalling, the prevailing culture did not encourage challenges to the way things were done and patient care was not prioritised. Leadership was ineffective. The report highlighted the need for a culture of honesty and openness, with an absolute priority given to the needs of the patients and protection of patients from harm. The Francis Report has continued to permeate the literature since it was published in 2013.

In the middle of the current pandemic crisis, the present government has announced new proposals to again change the NHS (UK Health and Care Bill, 2021). The stated aim of the current proposed change is to move power away from those who manage the NHS into the hands of the government. Power is to be centralised again, after all the efforts in the last policy changes to decentralise power. The key proposals for change are within NHS England, and include:

- Structural reform: The current 100 plus CCGs (Clinical Commissioning Groups) across the country will be replaced by 42–44 integrated care systems (ICSs) with the task of bringing all the systems together to plan and

commission health and social care. GPs, hospitals and local authorities will have Board responsibilities, with consultation with bodies such as social care and housing agencies. NHS England and NHS Improvement will merge.
- Collaboration and competition: The government wishes our views of competition within the NHS to change, there will no longer be an assumption that competition is the only means of bringing about improvement. However, the internal market will remain in the NHS, with distinct responsibilities for commissioners and providers. Patients will have the right to have their care undertaken by a private provider. The buzz word in the proposed changes is 'collaboration' with private providers and NHS organisations working together instead of competing. There will be an expectation of sharing of information between health and social care bodies with increased collaboration between ICSs and commissioners.
- Public health: The government proposes to give itself new powers in the arena of advertising unhealthy foods and the need for fluoridation of water.
- Safety: It is proposed that the health and safety investigation branch be underpinned by law and that ministers will have the power to intervene in professional regulation. It is proposed that there be a statutory medical examiner system within the NHS to scrutinise all deaths where a coroner is not involved.
- Social care: The Care Quality Commission will assess local authority delivery of adult social care and there will be new financial powers for the health secretary to include receiving data from all adult social care providers, to enable them to provide financial support as required, and the ability to impose capital spending limits on Foundation Trusts.

With these many changes in policy and government initiatives, is it any wonder that change attempts fail? The system has become more and more complex.

You might ask why have we focused our policy list here in this chapter on NHS England. It is because there have been so very many initiatives in England, far more than in the other three UK nations, without any apparent unifying strategy, illustrating the challenges of change for the workforce and the public. Molloy *et al.* (2016) found 179 such initiatives in the period from mid-June 2011 to December 2015 and associated this with a likelihood that it would lead to demotivation at the front line of health care delivery, with staff believing change is for change's sake rather than an expectation of improving quality.

By comparison, health policy direction in Scotland appears far more coherent (Dayan & Edwards, 2017). For example, the development of Clinical Standards Boards for Scotland in 1999, the development of Quality Improvement Scotland (QIS) from this in 2003, with initiatives such as the Scottish Patient Safety Programme within the QIS from 2008 and the Healthcare Environment Inspectorate started within QIS from 2009. Greater coherence than in England continued with publication of the Healthcare Quality Strategy in 2010, and the QIS becoming Healthcare Improvement Scotland in 2011 as it took over responsibility for inspecting private healthcare provision. The point that stands out is that the policy framework progresses within a much more unified overall strategy, with greater adherence to the underlying principles and values of the original NHS. This should mean that change is better received, the greater coherence engendering greater trust in policymakers. Robson (2019) identifies some 30 or more pieces of primary legislation related to health and social care since devolution in Scotland, and further secondary legislation but states the process has typically been one of 'gradual evolution' with considerable continuity. She singles out public health for making huge changes since devolution, with marked improvement in levels of cigarette smoking and alcohol consumption. Despite this, death rates have not improved in the most deprived communities and health inequalities are worsening.

In 2016, NHS Scotland introduced 31 Integration Authorities, partnerships between 14 NHS Boards and 32 local councils, designed to improve the integration between health and social care. The Accounts Commission, in its update (Accounts Commission, 2018), noted that there had been progress in some fields, for example there were less delays when discharging people from hospital and it was more likely that people at the end of their lives would spend time at home rather than in hospital. But to drive integration forward, the Accounts Commission noted the need for better strategic planning and overcoming barriers to enable the focus to be on improved outcomes for those in need. Collaborative leadership was recommended, and the importance of sharing relevant data with both staff and patients was emphasised. Better engagement between people and their communities and those leading the Integration Authorities was recommended, and the importance of being open and honest was stressed. The OECD (2016) also recommend that Healthcare Improvement Scotland relook at the potentially conflicting roles within this organisation, that of scrutiny and that of quality improvement. So even though policy has shown greater continuity in Scotland, there is much to do to improve the way change takes place.

The Healthcare Financial Management Association notes the huge changes which have occurred since the inception of the NHS in Wales in terms of legislation, structure, staff numbers, demographic of patients, funding and life expectancy. Highlighting the challenges faced, the HFMA (2018) notes that, despite the changes in policy, recent targets, set at 95%, have not been achieved for: duration in an emergency care facility (83.2%); time from referral to treatment (87.4%); being newly diagnosed with cancer and start of treatment (84%).

The top-down regulation which is a feature of NHS England is criticised by the OECD (2016) arguing that this leaves a void, with a lack of opportunity for local initiatives, so that health care staff feel unable to contribute meaningfully to problem solving and developing new ways of delivering care. Such a system has engendered distrust of those in power. Added to this are the many different national bodies, with little integration between them, despite the stated aim of improving quality. Opportunities for the workforce to initiate change is also needed in Scotland (OECD, 2016). Wales is praised for having such as system, but without the central power to drive changes through. Finding the balance between local initiatives and getting those which work into place and expanded across the country is still a challenge. NHS Northern Ireland is described as having clear systems for integration of health and social care in place, but a need for greater use of this to enable better individualised care (Davies & Mannion, 2013).

There have been some notable success stories, for example banning smoking in public places, with Scotland's earlier ban seeing earlier results in terms of reduced mortality from heart attacks (Greer, 2016). But it is difficult to make comparisons between the four countries of the UK since devolution. The OECD (2016) describes the energy put into improvements in health care quality and the high global reputation of many UK health policies, but the lack of evidence in the form of measurement of improvement in quality. They recommend better data, which would enable leaders of the health systems in the four countries of the UK to make comparisons, and discuss which policies are more successful. Greer (2016) also argues for data which are not only better than what is currently available, but also data which are able to be used for comparison between the four UK nations. He argues that politicians do not want such comparable data as this would expose the failings of policy. Connolly et al. (2010) undertook a review of performance of the four health care systems since devolution and noted how difficult it was to compare data, for example for waiting times, which were not measured in the same way. From the data available, they suggest that waiting times were better in England than in the other three countries, but that it was difficult to link expenditure to improved outcomes.

Policy changes to the NHS and the impact on quality, productivity, financial health of the NHS and the health of the nation

Despite the considerable resources given to change, there is limited statistical data on change success or change failure in health and social care. The evidence that is available, for example from comprehensive reviews of many of the UK Government's health care policies, points to limited successes of health care changes with limited benefits to patients, not much change in productivity and many financial challenges (Ham, 2014; Ham et al., 2015; Kings' Fund, 2011; Anandaciva et al., 2017; West & Dawson, 2012; Molloy et al., 2016; Accounts Commission, 2018). Analysis of the role of CCGs shows a mixed picture. Around 40% of CCGs are deemed to be failing, or at risk of failing, to discharge their functions (National Audit Office, 2018). The financial position of Trusts and CCGs show a pattern of poor health with the expectation that they will spend beyond their budget and half of CCGs' financial positions are in jeopardy and their overspending may be resolved either through deferring or annulling their accounts (Murray et al., 2017).

Most targets have not been met, or have been changed, or policy direction has changed so that the original target is meaningless (Palmer et al., 2020). For example, the Shared Delivery Plan, 2015–2020, promised 5000 more GPs, when in fact there has been a reduction of 1634 full time fully qualified permanent GPs since 2016; waiting time targets have not been met; less people have been referred to psychological therapies than expected; and the plan for digital health records is well behind schedule. If anything, the nations' health shows variation across the four countries and internationally, our health status does not match that of the EU, considering our wealth. Why then do these incessant policies continue? Another is imminent, however. A press release from the Nuffield Trust issued on 6 July 2021 (Edwards, 2021, p. 1) following the publication of the Health and Care Bill 2021–2022 states, in relation to the increased political power proposed 'The evidence of the past suggests this may lead to worse decisions, and they will come to regret it', and in relation to social care reform 'the social care reforms in this Bill do not solve any of the problems that have brought this sector to a point of crisis'.

We have referred to the nations' health earlier. There are variations across the four countries and internationally and our health status does not match that of the EU considering our wealth. Life expectancy and healthy life expectancy show a difference between the rich and the poor. In England, life expectancy for males is 83.5 years, for females 86.4 years for those from a higher socio-economic background. In deprived areas life expectancy for males is 74.1 years and for females it is 78.7 years. These differences are seen too in healthy life expectancy between the wealthy and the poor. People living in deprived areas can expect to be in poorer health longer compared to those in less deprived areas (male 21.8, 12.8 years and females 27.3, 15.3 years, respectively). On average, people living in the south of the country have better health outcomes than their counterparts elsewhere in the country. Within the four nations that make up the UK, there are also variations in health. In Scotland, life expectancy is falling and is the lowest across all UK countries. For females it is 81.1 years, for males it is 77.1 years. However, the variation is small between the other countries. For England, the average life expectancy for females is 82.7 years, for males it is 78.7 years. In Wales, for females it is 82.3 years, for males 78.3 years. In Northern Ireland, for females it is 82.3 years, for males 78.4 years. International comparison in 2019 showed male and female life expectancy across all UK countries to be below that of their counterparts in the EU (National Records of Scotland, 2020; Raleigh, 2021).

Further evidence of the health of the nation is examined in a recent report and paints a worrying picture of the health of the nation and remarks that 'the evidence we have reviewed has convinced us that things are indeed falling apart in the UK'. However, these researchers are optimistic and suggest that the situation can change with the government making the necessary 'changes to improve health, wealth and social well-being for all' (Hiam et al., 2020, p. 13). They cite: life expectancy at a standstill; increased infant mortality in deprived areas; growing inequalities between the wealthy and the poor; and a 'death of despair' in parts of the population between the age of 45 and 54 years (a concept that has been developed in the US and apply to the population there where people are dying from drug and alcohol over consumption, suicides and alcohol related diseases). According to the report, this 'phenomenon' is now present in the UK population (p. 10). Drug related deaths in Scotland have increased by a factor of 4.6 over the last two decades so that they are currently the highest in Europe and 3.5 times higher than the overall UK figure (National Records of Scotland, 2021).

Policy changes to the NHS and the impact on the health and wellbeing of employees

As the largest employer in Europe, the NHS not only has the job of delivering quality health care to its population across the acute, primary care and community sectors but it has to manage its vast number of staff from a range of disciplines who are providing care on a daily basis. Within primary care, there are a huge range of GP practices where the vast majority of the population receive healthcare. GPs are the gatekeepers to other services. NHS Foundation Trusts manage community healthcare for adults, mental health, child and learning disability. The NHS has to adhere to a range of professional regulations from different regulatory bodies and unions, the Health and Safety Executive and the CQC, alongside managing expectations from the public, from government and from employees. Nurses make up the largest professional group in the NHS, followed by doctors and a range of other professional groups such as therapists, radiographers, dieticians, counsellors and others. There are also large numbers of 'support' staff consisting of essential workers, together with technical, financial, administrative and other staff.

Management of employees is the role of individual Trusts and usually employees' contracts mean that they are accountable to their specific employer. With the constant changes in the NHS, employees have had to adjust to new and changing contracts, change in terms and conditions, change in management and change in employers. This creates a constant challenge to employees' professional roles and practice with employers making decisions around new ways of working for health professionals, changing their roles and responsibilities, imposing power relationships, challenging their professional autonomy and in many instances imposing their will on employees without adequate professional consultation.

So constant policy change has had potentially damaging effects on staff wellbeing. However, positive experiences of staff and their wellbeing are associated with improved quality, safety and patient outcomes, not just in the UK but in many countries across the globe (Lee et al., 2013). In effect happy, engaged and satisfied staff means improved patient outcomes. Early studies found a link between good human resources practices and positive health outcomes for patients (West et al., 2002; West et al., 2006). The Boorman Review showed a clear connection between staff health and wellbeing and outcomes such as absenteeism, staff turnover, patient satisfaction, patient mortality and infection rates (Boorman, 2009). Similarly, West et al. (2011) showed a significant association between staff experience, staff absenteeism, and patient satisfaction, patient mortality and performance indicators. Further studies show the same pattern, West and Dawson's 2012 study found associations between staff engagement and patient satisfaction, patient mortality, infection rates, Annual Health Check scores, staff absenteeism and turnover. A study by Powell et al. (2014) examined the effect of staff engagement and satisfaction on the performance of organisations with similar conclusions. Better staff experiences were linked to lower levels of absenteeism and greater patient satisfaction. They indicated that no one group of staff experience had more weight, but that nurses' experience had a greater bearing on absenteeism with medical and dental staff next. A recent report commissioned on behalf of NHS England found robust links between staff experience and patient satisfaction (Dawson, 2018). In the latest report on the same theme, Sizmur and Raleigh's (2018) found that poor staff experience was associated with increased sickness absence rates. Staff's wellbeing was being adversely affected due to insufficient staffing levels which often had to be covered by agency staff. Patient experiences, they indicated, are impacted by workforce factors with increased spending on agency staff, and fewer medical and nursing staff which results in fewer nurses per patient, and increased bed occupancy. They state (p. 3) these 'findings are unsurprising'. The employment of agency staff 'provides less continuity and stability of care, and inadequate staffing and high bed occupancy will impact negatively on the quality of inpatient care'. Thus, within the NHS, studies consistently show the association between better staff engagement and satisfaction and better patient experience and patient outcomes. And yet staff wellbeing has not been attended to.

The impact of constant change is seen for all professional groups in the NHS. The constant rise of workload has meant that health professionals have found it harder to develop therapeutic relationships with their patients as the pressure to discharge accelerates (Bunting, 2020). The continuous re-organisation and blame and fear culture have had a bearing on hospital doctors, GPs, nurses and other health professional groups' health and wellbeing, with a surge of professionals reporting to their unions and professional bodies and the stresses they are facing. The Kings' Fund has raised its concern as doctors are reporting low morale and GPs are reporting that they are unable to manage their workload (Baird *et al.*, 2016). GPs are leaving the profession so that the ratio fell from 65 GPs per 100,000 population in 2014 to 60 per 100,000 population in 2017 (Triggle, 2019) and Palmer (2019) identifies the considerable differences in numbers of GPs across the UK countries and across the regions of England. The changes in policy over time have seen GPs working longer hours, with increased administrative burdens placed on them. Policy changes have not placed value on the human side of medicine. Instead, money and metrics, measurable units based on cost, have been the focus. These are unable to capture the complex role which the GP undertakes.

The numerous and significant changes in the NHS have had an impact on the wellbeing of the workforce but this does not appear to have been acknowledged in research and advice. Kelly (2017) summarises the issues. For example, nurses are advised that there is an expectation for resilience and coping that goes with the job and having a healthy lifestyle is part of this (Kushner & Ruffin, 2015). Nursing is facing a recruitment crisis (RCN, 2018), with large numbers of posts unfilled, so being healthy is both necessary and expected to avoid absence through ill health and to ensure the aging workforce remain in post for longer. Being healthy is seen as a duty and a requirement for this professional group (While, 2014). In other words, these papers are stating that having a healthy lifestyle is a professional expectation. The leadership of nursing is suggesting that nurses need to take responsibility for their own health to practise safely and effectively, and maximise their positive impact on population health (NHS England, 2016). The International Council of Nurses (2010) suggested that nurses should eat healthily and exercise appropriately, and the NMC (2014) told nurses that role modelling is a statutory requirement. Nurses may thus feel blamed by those who should offer support. There is a lack of support for the pressures and stress they have been experiencing in an ever-changing NHS. There is no acknowledgement of the huge impact of constant and continuing change.

There is now a crisis in nursing; 17,000 nurses under the age of 40 left the NHS in 2016–2017. There has been an increase of 24% in the risk of suicide amongst female health care professionals, and according to the ONS (2017), this figure is due to the large numbers of high-risk suicides amongst nurses. Kester and Wei's (2018) literature review addressing strategies to promote nurse resilience points to a study by the Robert Wood Foundation, which found that 18% of nurses experience depression, a higher rate than the general public. The same literature review found that amongst nurses there is considerable dissatisfaction with the work they do and are expected to do. They experienced compassion fatigue, burnout, secondary trauma and the sheer volume of their work together with the emotional labour of caring had a negative impact on their personal and professional lives. Maybin et al. (2016) found that district nursing numbers have fallen and there is now a gap between service needs and numbers of district nurses. They conclude that this situation is affecting staff wellbeing resulting in 'poor morale', 'stress and fatigue' with the not surprising outcome that 'some staff are leaving'. There is a desire by nurses for employers to address job-related pressures (Kelly, 2017) and to support them to make positive lifestyle changes (Buchvold et al., 2015; Nahm et al., 2012). Doing so would support the nursing workforce to be in a better state of readiness for change.

So, the complexity of the health service, through constant and incessant policy change, has had a negative effect on the workforce. In turn, this has been linked to poorer patient outcomes.

Having introduced the ideas in this chapter, we take some time to consider the complexity of change in Chapter 2. We introduce the nature of health care change in the UK, summarising major policy changes which have occurred, the purposes of these changes and their effectiveness with reference to the nations' health, productivity, impact on the workforce and economic factors. The reasons for failure of many of the introduced changes are considered and the importance to the change process is emphasised. We identify that managing change is complex, especially in large organisations such as the NHS. Complexity is contributed to by culture, values, professional rivalries, financial constraints, political interference, incessant change through successive governments, a top-down management approach and a sense of size which means that individuals may feel voiceless. Power is not equally distributed and the expertise of those in clinical practice may not be listened to or valued. There are differences in culture not just across organisations, but across departments and units within the same organisation. Similarly, there are differences across the four nations of the UK, both in stated values, in policy and in practice.

The chapter proposes that successful change is possible in such large organisations, but change will only be effective if its focus is on the human dimension rather than on structures and processes.

Models and tools to support change management: cognition, emotion and behaviour

There is a plethora of organisational change management and behavioural approaches, models, theories and tools used to aid change management, but despite this the success rate of change in organisations has been universally at 30% (Beer & Nohria, 2000; Balogun & Hope Hailey, 2004), has not improved over the years (Rouse, 2011; Jacobs et al., 2013; Jansson, 2013; Michel et al., 2013) and has continued, including failure rates for change initiatives of up to 70% (Sackman et al., 2009; Burnes & Jackson, 2011; Burnes, 2017). With the relentless policy changes, successive governments have given enormous resources to managing change. National change agencies have been established and de-established and external consultancies commissioned, yet continue offering a gamut of ideas, theories, tools and advice on change management. However, there is no unified voice on successful change management nor any evaluation on how the process of change is managed nor any clear evidence of change success or failure.

We argue that successful change must consider human nature during the change process but most Change Management Models, theories and improvement tools do not consider the human element of change. Often a heavy focus is put on changing people's thinking only, dismissing the significance of the power of emotion, the impact of change on emotions and the benefits of addressing emotions during change. Together with this lack of consideration of human nature, practitioners face other vulnerabilities which pose a challenge for change. They experience high emotional labour of caring, work in inadequate conditions with lack of support, long working hours, experience burnout, high patient demand and high stress levels and are employed in large organisations with many complexities, the absence of a universal change formula and the absence of a unified voice on how best to manage change. These issues are considered in Chapter 5.

The reliance on models of change and improvement tools which only focus on changing thinking, a top-down change management approach, a focus on outcomes rather than people, is challenged in this book. It is argued that successful and sustainable change requires emotional and cognitive readiness for change which in turn creates preparedness of people for the change, thus making for a smoother and more effective implementation.

In Chapter 3, we provide a critique of current change management theories, models and approaches, focusing on planned change, emergent change, improvement tools and approaches specific to health care settings. This is important reading to support an understanding of the similarities and differences between approaches. We explore the work of Kurt Lewin which underpins many of the approaches to change used since 1950 and we explore the opportunity for success with the different elements of his work, and yet the way his work has been simplified to make it far less effective. Based on the work of Lewin, other models were developed and Kotter is used as an example of a planned approach to change. These step-by-step approaches tend towards the hierarchical management of change, with little emphasis on the complex situations in health care settings where change is occurring. There are elements of the importance of cognition in these models, in so far as the models identify the need to ensure the nature of the change is clearly articulated and explained. But there is very little evidence of understanding that change can have an emotional impact and little to engage the workforce in influencing change.

We also explore organisational development, which similarly had its roots in the work of Lewin. The early values of organisational development changed as time went by, and change started to be applied hierarchically to larger and larger organisations. Opportunities to engage with the workforce to effect meaningful and sustainable change were not evident, and instead of changing the way change was imposed, more changes were introduced using the same ineffective strategies.

We then look at theory related to emergent change. A different approach is needed here, as this kind of change is not foreseeable, it is more opportunistic in nature. A change in the environment or a change in world health or population may trigger situations in which the health service has to adapt without knowing how the end point of the change might appear. For change to be successful, leaders must have clear understanding of their workforce and the complex environment in which work takes place, and must be able to involve and listen to the workforce. An understanding of culture and values is needed by leaders and we begin to see the importance of organisational readiness for change. We finish Chapter 3 by exploring a number of approaches to change in health care settings in the UK and North America, some of which are based on planned approaches to change. We also consider improvement methodologies used for quality improvement.

There are models and theories of change that have a focus on emotion or on human behaviour and these are outlined in Chapter 4. Unfortunately, they do not typically also include the importance of cognition, nor the importance of readiness for change. We compare and contrast the key features, similarities and differences amongst these models and explore the philosophy and principles underpinning these models and theories, analysing them through the lens of human emotion, cognition and change. We argue that through the interconnectedness between emotion and cognition, cognitive and emotional readiness for change could be developed to aid successful change.

Through these two chapters (3 and 4), we show that most change models have been designed under the assumption that change management is best achieved through cognition, believing that successful change can only take place with changing people's thinking. We further argue that while there are models that can aid behaviour change, these tend to lack a focus on ensuring emotional and cognitive readiness for change. These models therefore miss the opportunity to assess readiness to ensure preparedness for the implementation of change. Thus, models either typically focus on thinking only, emotion only or behaviour change.

We demonstrate that change, be it organisational, clinical practice, education, large or small scale – whether in health care, education or other organisations – generates mostly negative emotions and has a serious impact on the health and wellbeing of health care professionals, as well as high cost to health care organisations. We show how negative and positive emotions about change need to be acknowledged and understood, especially in professional groups that have high emotional labour, and if addressed can contribute to successful change management in health and social care settings.

We also illuminate the role and importance of employers in addressing the wellbeing of employees, in particular the emotional impact of the job of caring. Moreover, we highlight that top executive and management needs a cultural shift around enacting change towards new models of leadership and shared leadership, valuing people at all levels in the organisation, empowerment of all, emotional intelligence across senior teams, engaging and involving staff at all levels, developing a culture of innovation and a clear focus on change for the betterment of patients not just for financial probity.

It will be no surprise therefore to find a number of chapters in this book which include elements of emotion; Chapters 5–7 consider different aspects of emotion and change. We explore the nature of emotion and how it impacts judgement and reasoning. We identify that change impacts the individual physically, emotionally, psychologically and financially, and can lead to many health effects and even disability. This is not a state conducive to successful change, quite the opposite, such a state creates resistance to change. The nature of emotional labour is examined. We argue that the nature of caring already takes an emotional toll on these professionals. Change brings an additional emotional burden and this needs to be given serious consideration when any change is proposed. Understanding and acknowledging the emotions of the workforce who will have to enact change can support positive and sustained change. The way in which change agents acknowledge emotion can benefit or stifle change. Change agents who take a negative view of human nature may blame employee resistance for a failure of change to take place, rather than considering emotion as an aspect of change management.

Emotional and cognitive readiness for change

People bring about change, and focusing on people rather than processes enables consideration of emotional and cognitive readiness for change. In Chapter 6, we explore the concept of readiness for change and how it can be applied to the context where changes are occurring. Change readiness is fundamental, without this readiness change is unlikely to be successful because change requires individuals to understand the rationale for the change, adjust and adapt themselves emotionally and cognitively to new processes, structures, people, policies and new ways of working. Consideration of emotional and cognitive elements in change management are aspects of this concept of readiness for change and we argue that through the acknowledgement of an interconnectedness between emotion and cognition, a model of readiness for change could be very valuable in bringing about successful change and we introduce such an approach through the AC-W Change Management Model and its accompanying tool. In Chapter 7, we discuss the AC-W Change Management Model which considers people's feeling and thinking, and we illuminate how this model can help towards emotional and cognitive readiness for change which could provide the energy, motivation and engagement needed for change.

We have chapters on application of theory. We met with colleagues experiencing different kinds of change and in a variety of settings. In Chapters 8 and 9, we discuss the model in practice, on its own and in conjunction with Lewin and Kotter's models, using case studies drawn from organisational and practice changes across a variety of settings including acute; primary care and community; mental health; children's services; as well as personal changes with clients. Real case studies from the field help to illustrate how change in clinical practice, organisational change and other kinds of change can be managed retrospectively, in real time or prospectively. Assessing emotional and cognitive readiness for change provides details of the impact of change on practitioners, their needs, and the resources and preparation required for enacting any change. The results once analysed can be used to construct a preparedness and implementation plan for emotional and cognitive readiness for change thus contributing to effective change.

Summary

Health policy in the UK has changed frequently and continues to change. This has led to changes in structure and delivery of health services. Such constant change, often lacking coherence, has caused the workforce to become weary and sceptical of change. This chapter has summarised our case for new thinking on change management. We have outlined the obstacles to and significant factors involved in ensuring successful change. The challenge to successful change is huge.

The old ways of managing change in healthcare are not proving effective. We are suggesting that with the sheer volume of incessant health care policies, political interference from successive governments, little or no improvement in the nations' health, the negative impact on the wellbeing of staff, a culture of directive top-down approach to leadership, a health service in constant debt, change models, improvement tools and theories that treat people as machines are all inhibitors to effective change. Successful change requires new thinking. People are the greatest resource and strength in the NHS, and these current conditions do not lend themselves to ensuring employees' emotional and cognitive readiness for change, which is potentially the key to successful change management.

Change leaders need to put the focus on people, human nature, recognising that the job of caring itself already takes a huge emotional toll on healthcare professionals, and change is an added emotional burden. The AC-W Change Management

Model focuses on emotional and cognitive readiness for change, recognising that these two interactive and interdependent elements are necessary to manage change successfully. Assessing emotional and cognitive readiness for change offers the opportunity for staff to become engaged and involved in voicing their professionalism and thus creating a preparedness programme for change that is more meaningful and relevant to them and the service they are providing, the setting in which they are working and the peers they will be collaborating with. Such a programme is likely to reflect their professional role, create the much-needed energy and motivation required for change, thus ensuring successful change through emotional and cognitive readiness for change.

References

Accounts Commission, 2018. *Health and Social Care Integration. Update on Progress.* Edinburgh: Audit Scotland. Available at: www.audit-scotland.gov.uk/uploads/docs/report/2018/nr_181115_health_socialcare_update.pdf

Anandaciva, S., Jabbal, J., Maguire, D., & Chijoko, L., 2017. *Quarterly Monitoring Report 24.* Kings' Fund. Available at: kingsfund.org.uk

Baird, B., Charles, A., Honeyman, M., Maguire, D., & Das, P., 2016. *Understanding Pressures in General Practice.* London: The Kings' Fund.

Balogun, J., & Hope Hailey, V., 2004. *Exploring Strategic Change* (2nd ed.). London: Prentice Hall.

Beer, M., & Nohria, N., 2000. *Breaking the Code of Change.* Boston, MA: Harvard Business Review Press.

Boorman, S., 2009. *NHS Health and Well-being Review.* Leeds: Department of Health.

Buchvold, H., Pallesen, S., Øyane, N., & Bjorvatn, B., 2015. 'Associations between night work and BMI, alcohol, smoking, caffeine and exercise: A cross-sectional study'. *BMC Public Health*, 15: 1112. https://doi.org/10.1186/s12889-015-2470-2

Bunting, M., 2020. *Labours of Love.* London: Granta Publications.

Burnes, B., 2017. *Managing Change* (7th ed.). Harlow: Pearson.

Burnes, B., & Jackson, P., 2011. 'Success and failure in organizational change: An exploration of the role of values'. *Journal of Change Management*, 11(2): 133–162.

Connolly, S., Bevan, G., & Mays, N., 2010. *Funding and Performance of Healthcare Systems in the Four Countries of the UK before and after Devolution.* London: Nuffield Trust.

Davies, H., & Mannion, R., 2013. 'Will prescriptions for cultural change improve the NHS?'. *BMJ*, 346: 1–4.

Dawson, J., 2018. *Links between NHS Staff Experience and Patient Satisfaction: Analysis of Surveys from 2014 and 2015.* London: NHS England.

Dayan, M., & Edwards, N., 2017. *Learning from Scotland's NHS.* London: Nuffield Trust. Available at: www.nuffieldtrust.org.uk/files/2017-07/learning-from-scotland-s-nhs-final.pdf

Edwards, N., 2021. *Nuffield Trust Response to Health and Care Bill.* London: Nuffield Trust. Available at: www.nuffieldtrust.org.uk/news-item/nuffield-trust-response-to-health-and-care-bill

Francis, R., 2013. *Report of the Mid Staffordshire NHS Foundation Trust Public Inquiry.* London: The Stationery Office.

Greer, S., 2016. 'Devolution and health in the UK: Policy and its lessons since 1998'. *British Medical Bulletin*, 118(1): 16–24. https://doi.org/10.1093/bmb/ldw013

Ham, C., 2014. *Improving NHS Care by Engaging Staff and Devolving Decision-making. Report of the Review of Staff Engagement and Empowerment in the NHS.* London: The King's Fund.

Ham, C., Baird, B., Gregory, S., Jabbal, J., & Alderwick, H., 2015. *The NHS Under the Coalition Government. Part One: NHS Reform*. London: King's Fund.

HFMA Briefing, 2018. *70 Years of the NHS in Wales: The Changing Role of the NHS Finance Function*. Bristol: HFMA. Available at: www.hfma.org.uk/docs/default-source/publications/Briefings/70-years-of-the-nhs-in-wales.pdf?sfvrsn=df466fe7_0

Hiam, L., Dorling, D., & McKee, M., 2020. 'Things fall apart: The British Health Crisis 2010–2020'. *British Medical Bulletin*, 1–12. Available at: https://academic.oup.com/bmb/advance-article/doi/10.1093/bmb/ldz041/5812717

International Council of Nurses, 2010. *Delivering Quality, Serving Communities: Nurses Leading Chronic Care*. Geneva: ICN. Available at: ghdonline.org

Jacobs, G., van Witteloostuijn, A., & Christe-Zeyse, J., 2013. 'A theoretical framework of organizational change'. *Journal of Organizational Change Management*, 26(5): 772–792.

Jansson, N., 2013. 'Organizational change as practice: A critical analysis'. *Journal of Organizational Change Management*, 26(6): 1003–1019.

Kelly, M., 2017. 'Should nurses be expected to role model healthy lifestyles to patients?'. *Nursing Times*, 113(10): 46–48.

Kester, K., & Wei, H., 2018. 'Building nurse resilience'. *Nursing Management*, 49(6): 42–45.

Kings' Fund, 2011. *How is the NHS Performing? Quarterly Monitoring Report*. London: Kings' Fund.

Kushner, J., & Ruffin, T., 2015. 'Empowering a healthy practice environment'. *Nursing Clinics of North America*, 50(1): 167–183.

Lee, R.T., Seo, B., Hladkyj, S., Lovell, B.L., & Schwartzmann, L., 2013. 'Correlates of physician burnout across regions and specialties: A meta-analysis'. *Human Resources for Health*, 11: 48). Available at: biomedcentral.com

Maybin, J., Charles, A., & Honeyman, M., 2016. *Understanding Quality in District Nursing Services*. London: King's Fund. Available at: quality_district_nursing_aug_2016.pdf (kingsfund.org.uk)

Michel, A., By, R., & Burnes, B., 2013. 'The limitations of dispositional resistance in relation to organizational change'. *Management Decision*, 51(4): 761–780.

Molloy, A., Martin, S., Gardner, T., & Leatherman, S., 2016. *A Clear Road Ahead: Creating a Coherent Quality Strategy for the English NHS*. London: The Health Foundation.

Murray, R., Jabbal, J., Thompson, J., Baird, B., & Maguire, D., 2017. *Quarterly Monitoring Report 23*. London: The King's Fund. Available at: kingsfund.org.uk

Nahm, E.-S., Warren, J., Zhu, S., An, M., & Brown, J., 2012. 'Nurses' self-care behaviors related to weight and stress'. *Nursing Outlook*, 60(5): e23–31.

National Audit Office, 2018. *A Review of the Role and Costs of Clinical Commissioning Groups*. London: NAO.

National Records of Scotland, 2020. *Life Expectancy in Scotland*. Edinburgh: National Records of Scotland. Available at: nrscotland.gov.uk

National Records of Scotland, 2021. *Life Expectancy in Scotland*. Edinburgh: National Records of Scotland. Available at: nrscotland.gov.uk

NHS England, 2016. *Leading Change, Adding Value*. A framework for nursing, midwifery and care staff. NHS England. Available at: https://www.england.nhs.uk/wp-content/uploads/2016/05/nursing-framework.pdf

Nursing and Midwifery Council, 2014. *Standards for Competence for Registered Nurses*. London: NMC.

OECD, 2016. *OECD Reviews of Health Care Quality: United Kingdom 2016*. Paris: OECD Publishing. Available at: www.oecd.org/unitedkingdom/oecd-reviews-of-health-care-quality-united-kingdom-2016-9789264239487-en.htm

ONS (Office for National Statistics), 2017. *Suicide by occupation, England: 2011 to 2015*. Available at: https://www.ons.gov.uk/peoplepopulationandcommunity/birthsdeathsandmarriages/deaths/articles/suicidebyoccupation/england2011to2015

Palmer, B., Buckingham, H., Crellin, N., & Oung, C., 2020. *Hindsight 2020: Lessons on Setting Targets in Health and Social Care*. Briefing. London: Nuffield Trust. Available at: www.nuffieldtrust.org.uk/research/hindsight-2020-lessons-on-setting-targets-in-health-and-social-care

Palmer, W., 2019. 'Is the number of GPs falling across the UK?'. *Nuffield Trust blog*, 8 May.

Powell, M., Dawson, J., Topakas, A., Durose, J., & Fewtrell, C., 2014. 'Staff satisfaction and organisational performance: Evidence from a longitudinal secondary analysis of the NHS staff survey and outcome data'. *Health Services and Delivery Research*, 2(50): 1–336.

Raleigh, V., 2021. *What is Happening to Life Expectancy in England?* London: The King's Fund. Available at: kingsfund.org.uk

RCN, 2018. *NHS Reveals Staffing Crisis in New Recruitment Figures*. Online news item. London: Royal College of Nursing. Available at: rcn.org.uk

Robson, K., 2019. 'Has devolution been good for our health?' *Blog Post*. Edinburgh: SPICe. Available at: https://spice-spotlight.scot/2019/03/04/has-devolution-been-good-for-our-health/

Rouse, W., 2011. 'Necessary competencies for transforming an enterprise'. *Journal of Enterprise Transformation*, 1(1): 71–92.

Sackman, S., Eggenhofer-Rehart, P., & Friesl, M., 2009. 'Sustainable change: Long term effects towards developing a learning organization'. *Journal of Applied Behavioural Science*, 45: 521–549.

Sizmur, S., & Raleigh, V., 2018. *The Risks to Care Quality and Staff Wellbeing of an NHS System Under Pressure*. Oxford: Picker Institute Europe.

Triggle, N., 2019. 'GP pressure: Numbers show first sustained drop for 50 years'. *BBC News*.

UK Parliament, 2021. *Health and Care Bill*. London: House of Commons. Available at: https://bills.parliament.uk/bills/3022/publications

West, M., Borrill, C., Dawson, J., Scully, J., Carter, M., Anelay, S., & Waring, J., 2002. 'The link between the management of employees and patient mortality in acute hospitals'. *International Journal of Human Resource Management*, 13(8): 1299–1310.

West, M., & Dawson, J., 2012. *Employee Engagement and NHS Performance*. London: Kings Fund. Available at: Employee engagement and NHS performance (kingsfund.org.uk)

West, M., Dawson, J., Admasachew, L., & Topakas, A., 2011. *NHS Staff Management and Health Service Quality*. Lancaster: Lancaster University Management School and the Work Foundation Aston Business School.

West, M., Guthrie, J., Dawson, J., Borrill, C., & Carter, M., 2006. 'Reducing patient mortality in hospitals: The role of human resource management'. *Journal of Organizational Behavior*, 27(7): 983–1002.

While, A., 2014. 'Are nurses fit for their public health role?'. *International Journal of Nursing Studies*, 51(9): 1191–1194.

2
COMPLEXITY AND CHANGE MANAGEMENT

Introduction

We refer to complexity on a number of occasions in this book. The NHS is the largest employer in Europe, but it is not just this large size which is a challenge for change, it is the many and varied components which it now comprises and the impact this has on its function. Factors at play which affect change include culture and values, professional rivalries, incessant change by successive governments with political interference, financial constraints, unequal distribution of power and a top-down management approach.

The complexity of the current NHS is captured by Sturgeon (2014, p. 405) describing its transformation from a 'single national healthcare provider to a complex conglomeration of national and private organisations providing healthcare under the umbrella of the NHS brand'. The Kings Fund, in their alternative guide to NHS England, highlights this complexity in a YouTube clip (The Kings Fund, 2017). In this chapter, we include a consideration of values and culture and provide background to the complex system which is the NHS. But it would be wrong to think that NHS England is the same as the NHS in the other three countries which make up the UK. We address some of these differences and the challenges they pose for change.

The complexity of the NHS is complicated by the increased number of professional groups, each with their regulatory bodies, which identify values and culture within their professions. While the declared values of the different regulatory bodies are very similar, some of the ways in which professionals work together are complex, with issues of power and structural hierarchy giving rise to challenges.

A major issue related to complexity is the large number of policy changes that have occurred, with successive governments imposing structural changes which have impacted on the ability of the health professionals to do their work in a way which is compatible with their professional values. However, politicians have not been answerable for the ongoing challenges which the NHS has faced. We provide an overview of some of these changes, the stated aims and the resultant issues.

We propose that successful change is possible in a large organisation such as the NHS, whether it be practice, clinical or organisational change. Change does not need to equate to chaos, it can be better managed through listening to and working with the health professionals who strive daily to improve the health of the nation.

Culture

Organisational culture 'consists of the values, beliefs and assumptions shared by occupational groups' (Davies & Mannion, 2013, p. 1) which become established in patterns of behaviour and become evident as ways of working across the organisation. As Vincent (2010, p. 271) puts it: culture is 'how we do things round here'. However, the culture of professional caring can find itself at odds with business methods and a focus on cost saving.

In the UK health care sector, the negative impact of culture was highlighted by the Francis report in 2013. Poor culture was identified by this report as instrumental in the failures of care at Mid Staffordshire NHS Foundation Trust and the report highlighted the need for comprehensive change in this culture. While the report was based on the inquiry at Mid Stafford, poor culture was much more widespread across the NHS. Francis (2013) described a number of issues at play which impacted negatively on culture, including bullying, the priority of targets, poor engagement between management and staff, poor staff morale, feelings of isolation, lack of openness and honesty, overlooking poor behaviour, relying on external judgements rather than internal ones and denial of the existence of problems. A change in organisational culture was required, and the elements of this new culture were identified as: safety, ensuring no harm is done and aiming for excellent care; care, commitment and compassion; prioritising the needs of the patient; supporting empathy; providing assistance to patients; listening to patients; collaborative working; and escalating concerns to those who can support resolutions. It is shocking to think that such elements may not be part and parcel of a health care organisation's culture, but Francis stated that we must not be complacent, we must not assume a positive culture in our health care system. This is an important message if we are considering implementing change, the culture may not be as expected.

Since 2002, UK Government policy for health has driven forward a competitive environment within the NHS. When the NHS was established in 1948, the notion of health care consumers was not envisaged but over time this has changed. Sturgeon (2014, p. 409) provides a useful summary of the rise of neoliberalism, from the Thatcher years of entrepreneurialism and marketisation, not only within the wider economy but also within the public sector, with the health sector being seen to focus on 'competition and consumer power' by 1989. This move to consumerism and competition was later developed under the Blair government as a partnership between public, voluntary and private health care sectors, but with the emphasis on marketisation and the importance of the private sector. Today, people who require healthcare in the UK are considered as consumers, and the NHS is in the business of this consumption. Health care contracts are commercial opportunities for both state-run and private providers. Sturgeon (2014, p. 406) explains this in terms of commodification, a move from a non-commercial system to one of goods and services being 'both marketable and sought-after', a move to consumerism and competition. In a recent report, The Guardian outlined the share volume of money taken out of the NHS. In 2010, 8.4 billion was spent and by 2020, it rose to 14.4 billion, showing a 72% rise. From this sum, the private sector was accorded some 9.7 billion for providing a number of services (Campbell, 2021).

An extensive study of senior managers in English NHS hospital trusts (Mannion et al., 2009) demonstrated a change in their culture over the period 2001–2008. Using the Competing Values Framework, the researchers were able to compare managers' values at the start of the period to those at the end of the period. They found a change from what they call 'clan' culture (a more participative, relationship-based, culture with a focus on spontaneity and flexibility) at the start of the study to a more 'rational' culture (based on mechanistic processes, control and competition) by the end of the study. They highlighted the fact that this change in values of managers influenced the places in which health professionals worked. They recommended further research about how this might impact the experiences of patients, clinical outcomes and the professionalism of the staff.

By 2014, in a report for The King's Fund, Ham (2014) stated that the move to this rational style culture had gone too far, with 'targets and performance management, inspection and regulation, and competition and choice' (p. 3) being far too dominant, at the expense of more clan-based approaches to improvements from within the organisation. While Ham does not refer directly to the language of the Competing Values Framework, his messages are clear. The domination of competition has not benefited the culture of the NHS. He recommends greater valuing of 'innovation and experimentation' and clinical leadership, a change to 'collective and distributed' leadership and a less top-down approach to management (Ham, 2014, p. 4). Bunting (2020) meanwhile describes how responses to the Francis report focused too much on money and throughput, and not enough value was put on the role of caring. An interesting recent development from the Royal College of Nursing is the launch of Nursing Workforce Standards, aiming to set expectations of employers so that care delivery can be safe and effective. The need for such standards suggests that there are current challenges in the workplace to safe and effective delivery of nursing care.

Other authors highlight the complexity of culture within an organisation such as the NHS. Davies and Mannion (2013) are critical of some of the Francis report's recommendations, suggesting that some are aspirational rather than realistic, and identifying a lack of use of research evidence about how to shape positive cultural change. They challenge the recommendations, criticising the underlying assumptions that culture can be assessed and the parts linked to good care identified and deliberately changed; that change will lead inevitably to a better culture and better care; and that any such change in culture will be cost effective. These authors identify the 'large and distributed' system which is the NHS and the presumption which Francis makes of a common culture being both 'possible and desirable'. In fact, Scott *et al.* (2003) went so far as to argue that the relationship between organisational culture and health care effectiveness is unclear and Davies and Mannion (2013, p. 1) argue that the relation between culture and practice is much more 'complex and nuanced'. So, if change in culture is to occur, the complexity of such culture and the ill-defined relationship to performance should be acknowledged.

Challenging the view that organisational cultures are uniform, Morgan and Ogbonna (2008) carried out research in two large NHS Trusts in one Regional Health Authority in the UK, studying the variation in 'values, norms and assumptions' (p. 39) between doctors, nurses and non-clinical managers. Their study occurred at a time following the introduction of the notion of 'Clinical Governance' by the UK Labour Party in 1998, with a drive to improve standards through better leadership, better communication and better working across multidisciplinary teams, in other words, at a time when there was a drive for a change in culture in the NHS. Morgan and Ogbonna (2008) found that there was some agreement between different professional groups about their view of the philosophy of the NHS, that the main focus for provision of care should be individual need, not availability of funds. There was also agreement about the negative impact of government through imposition of constant new and untested interventions, many of which had proved to be unsuccessful (a view supported by the King's Fund study by Ham in 2014). The authors report their participants as hopeful of less government control, because the numerous and often disjointed policies had not had positive impact.

But apart from these two areas of agreement, there was diversity in the culture between the groups studied. For example, nursing groups were generally positive about the potential of the change to empower them and begin to address a perceived imbalance in power between professional groups, although they expressed concern about the cost of implementation, whereas medical staff were generally negative about the potential for benefit and about the lack of consultation. Areas of difference between professional groups appeared to be based on characteristics of that group, for example the tendency of medical staff to be more individualistic and of nursing staff to be more team based. Morgan and Ogbonna (2008) argue that culture within large organisations is multi-layered, operating at a variety of subcultural levels. They suggest that cultural agreement may only be possible across more wide-ranging goals. Davies and Mannion (2013) highlight that diversity of cultures operating within different parts of an organisation such as the NHS is to be expected and that even where common language is used to describe values, the language may be understood differently by different staff groups. The Francis report (2013) argues that while a large organisation may aspire to a common culture, this is unlikely to occur in such a complex system as the NHS, where culture is likely to vary between health care organisations and departments within these organisations. But while difference might occur, Francis argues, there is a fundamental need for a positive culture.

Work by Marshall et al. (2003) explored two very different cultural styles of management in Primary Care Trusts (PCTs). In hierarchical structures, the style was generally directive, driven by a political agenda, imposing change without reference to the existing culture, whereas in organisations described as having a clan-type culture, the style used for leadership was to fit in with the culture of the general practice and work with this to effect change. While there is no 'one size fits all' model for cultural change, a literature review by Willis et al. (2016) found six guiding principles when making sustainable culture change in an organisation. A common element amongst these principles is better integration of the workforce in making decisions for change and in carrying out such change, with distributed leadership. They recommend specific planning for the likely impact of change on clinical care and on those staff dealing directly with the public, supporting small changes towards a larger change, acknowledging the existing culture and the importance of collaborative interpersonal relationships. Reflecting on changes to SHAs and regions, a Nuffield Trust report states that 'The leadership style of the CEO influences the character of the organisation but, where a region has its own existing culture or approach, it will be easier if there is a good fit between the two' (Edwards & Buckingham, 2020, p. 25) suggesting that when appointing to senior positions this 'fit' of culture should be considered.

Effective and enduring change must be consistent with the existing culture (Carroll & Quijada, 2003), building on the strengths of this in order to move forward. This focus on the human dimension rather than just on structure and processes can form a part of ensuring readiness for change in a complex organisation.

Values

We identify values as part of culture, but also note that large organisations may hope for a common culture across their different groups and sections.

The NHS Constitution for England (2021), first published in 2012, includes lists of aspirational values associated with the NHS. These include putting patients first, valuing every individual, speaking out against poor practice, respect and dignity, listening to concerns and feedback, commitment to quality, striving for improvement, maximising use of resources. Similar values can be found on the NHS websites for the other UK countries, with NHS Scotland identifying the four values of: care and compassion; dignity and respect; openness, honesty and responsibility; and quality and teamwork (NHS Scotland, 2013). These are values one would expect in relation to a national health service and demonstrate an overarching aspiration for a common culture based on these shared values, but we want to draw out some of the particular challenges for change faced by the NHS in relation to values.

The different values evident in the NHS across the four different countries of the UK were the subject of a report by the Nuffield Trust in 2008 (Greer &

Rowland, 2008). Although the NHS began as a UK wide organisation, devolution in the late 20th century meant that policy difference was possible in different parts of the UK. The devolved National Health Services of England, Scotland, Wales and Northern Ireland are distinctive, with different embedded values. While recognising that stated values and actual values in practice may not be the same, the report noted the divergence of values within the four nations, with values in Scotland and Wales being centred on 'collaboration and collectivism' and 'communication and collectivism', respectively, and values in Northern Ireland being identified with 'democratic participation, neutrality and the new public health: having a say rather than having a choice' (p. 11). The authors note the stark contrast with the 'markets and technical solutions' which appear to be overarching values in NHS England.

Klein (2008) describes how the NHS in England has moved from a 'church' model, somewhat paternalistic, based on need, founded in trust, to a 'garage' model, based on consumer demand, choice and contracts. However, Klein points out that neither the original 1946 legislation which brought about the NHS, nor the 1979 Royal Commission on the NHS, were centred around statements of values. Values at an abstract, overarching level within Europe are identified as 'universality, access to good quality care, equity and solidarity' (Klein, 2008, p. 23) and as such they are difficult to criticise. He does criticise the fashion for value statements as equivalent to mission statements or organisational ambitions, arguing that such statements are not useful to practise but merely 'managerial fads' (Klein, 2008, p. 24). The explosion of such statements is posited as necessary because so much change in the health service means the underpinning values cannot be assumed.

Such value statements, generated at a managerial level, are often in competition with the values of the different health professional groups within NHS England. But this imposition of values cannot be said of NHS Scotland. Kerr and Feeley (2008) argue that the principles on which the NHS was based at its outset in 1946 are still evident in health care policy in Scotland. They describe the process of consultation across Scotland before the changes in the Fair to All policy were implemented, with the full and robust embracing of these original NHS principles by the people of Scotland, but the strong rejection of the idea that the private sector should be used by the NHS, because it went against these principles. Kerr and Feeley (2008) further argue that the National Framework for Service Change in Scotland (NFSCS), which was looking to make NHS Scotland future-proof, continued to reinforce the original principles, while making the service more patient-centred, easier to access and more collaborative, with a greater focus on quality and collectivism. The difference between 'collaboration' between professionals and patient is distinguished from merely offering a 'choice of options' to the patient. The report resulting from the NFSCS reflected the views of the Scottish public, who had the opportunity to attend town hall meetings, and who had been vociferous in their responses to the proposed change. There is a sense that the Scottish public have had greater input into the development of health policy in Scotland, particularly in the rejection of the market drivers of health which have been embraced in England.

This is not to say that the health professionals within the NHS in England have lost the original values of the NHS, rather that the policy framework within which they work has changed focus to consumers and markets. The concern for conflicts of interest based on 'personal, financial or commercial interests, incentives, targets or similar measures' (NMC, 2017, p. 1) prompted the release of a joint statement in 2017 by the Nursing and Midwifery Council (NMC), the Health and Care Professions Council (HCPC) and the General Medical Council along with the other six regulatory bodies under the Professional Standards Authority. This action clearly identifies that the professional values held by health professionals may differ from the values inherent in some of the environments in which they work.

Dayan and Edwards (2017, p. 3) identify that 'Scotland has a unique system of improving the quality of health care. It focuses on engaging the altruistic professional motivations of frontline staff to do better, and building their skills to improve'. The involvement of front-line staff in making changes means that the measures used are understood by those putting changes in place. Comparison is made to the English NHS, where changes initiated at the top of the organisation do not become enacted in clinical practice. This focus on the professionalism and trustworthiness of staff appears to extend throughout the health service in Scotland where consistency in structure over many years has enabled personal connections between senior appointees within the NHS. Similarly, the consistent approach appears to have led to consistency in focus on patient outcomes. Criticising changes in the structure of health services in England, a recent Nuffield Trust report recommends that 'The top team nationally needs to be of a manageable size and have high levels of trust and collegiate working' (Edwards & Buckingham, 2020, p. 25), something which is much more apparent in Scotland.

More praise for Scotland's system comes in the way that changes have been made within a consistent framework of quality improvement which has not been distracted by changes in the political situation. Dayan and Edwards (2017, p. 8) see this as in 'marked contrast' to the situation in England and Wales, where the overall plan has been changed frequently, with successive governments redesigning the health service or changing the priorities underlying health policy. The structure of the Scottish NHS is far less hierarchical than that in England and there appears to be greater integration and communication between government departments and those in charge of the health boards. This is not to say that it is plain sailing in Scotland. Financial pressures, the geography of the country and the need for inclusion of very rural communities, alongside the changing political situation, continue to provide significant challenges.

In Wales, Michael and Tanner (2008) argue that support for the original principles of the NHS remains evident and that these principles are well embedded in Welsh values, perhaps strengthened by the fact that Aneurin Bevan, a Welshman, founded the NHS on the workings of a medical aid society based in Tredegar in South Wales. The different health circumstances in Wales are also noted, with traditionally higher levels of poverty and the associated increased mortality impacting policy and providing particular challenges to devolution of health care. The commitment to a collective approach, with strong communication, appear as important values for NHS Wales. Longley (2015) comments that the change of pace in Wales is exceedingly slow despite policies which appear to be fundamentally sound. While Wales shares the financial challenges faced by the other three countries in the UK, it also faces the challenge of being a largely rural and in many cases deprived community, for example, the challenge of keeping its GPs. Welsh health policy has been driving for increased focus on prevention and less emphasis on hospital care.

Devolution of health policy was welcomed by Northern Ireland, to enable health policy to serve its largely rural communities, which differed greatly from other parts of the UK and from those of England in particular (Campbell, 2008). The political structures of Northern Ireland have provided unique challenges in supporting progress and change in health care provision. Campbell reiterates the inherent principles of the NHS as part of the values of Northern Ireland but these values have extended to include the value of 'nothing about me, without me'. That is, there is a real drive for people to have a say in health, whether within their immediate community or at regional level. There is also a drive for greater equity in health service provision and for improved public health. The drive in Northern Ireland since devolution has been focused on reducing the need for hospitals and centralising particular services; prevention of disease and promotion of health. Dayan and Heenan (2019) point out that during the last 20 years, there have been major reviews of health policy on seven occasions but with limited effective change. Using the Competing Values Framework, they mapped the culture in the Northern Ireland health care system and categorised it as more controlled than in the other three countries of the UK, pointing out that change is more likely to succeed if the system is more flexible. The authors highlight the opportunities for major change afforded by a system where the power is concentrated rather than distributed, but warn that this approach is likely to reduce flexibility in leadership to implement changes, which means that cultural tensions can occur. Enabling the workforce to offer practical and clinical solutions for change based in experience will be stamped out with a concentrated system of power. Dayan and Heenan (2019) warn that the system in England is in danger of mimicking this concentration of power, and that this is likely to be detrimental to a culture of change.

The differences in culture and size between the four nations means that what works in one country does not necessarily work well in another. However, some of the challenges experienced by England could be improved by reducing the inherent hierarchy of the health care system and providing a consistent rather than fragmented approach to quality improvement. The way in which the health boards in Scotland work to see through improvement is identified by Dayan and Edwards (2017) as a possible approach to use in Wales, where the structure is in place but a mechanism is needed to drive change forward, especially given the success of initiatives such as the 1000 lives improvement plan in Wales.

So, while there are shared values across the National Health Services of the four nations of the UK, there are also differences, and these have grown since devolution. Differences such as these can impact on how change is conceived and enacted. We now turn to consideration of the values of some of the health professions as evidenced in their regulatory bodies.

The values of each of the health professions are embedded in codes and standards of conduct. For example, the NMC which regulates the nursing and midwifery professions in the UK has a code of professional standards of practice and behaviour (NMC, 2015). The standards include prioritising people, practising effectively, preserving safety, and promoting professionalism and trust. The regulatory body for many other health professions is the HCPC. The standards of conduct performance and ethics detail the need to:

> promote and protect the interests of service users and carers; communicate appropriately and effectively; work within the limits of their knowledge and skills; delegate appropriately; respect confidentiality; manage risk; report concerns about safety; be open when things go wrong; be honest and trustworthy; and keep records of their work.
>
> *(HCPC, 2016, p. 1)*

Similarly, the General Medical Council (GMC, 2013) publish 'Good Medical Practice' which encompasses values and professionalism including knowledge, skills and performance; safety and quality; communication, partnership and teamwork; and maintaining trust. These different codes and standards act as a regulatory framework for the different professions, so that the health professional who does not uphold the standards could be potentially struck off their register and prohibited from working. It is clear from the above examples that the stated values from the regulatory bodies are very similar. The shared values are also evident in initiatives such as the six Cs of care, compassion, competence, communication, courage and commitment. These six Cs were identified first in nursing (Department of Health, 2012), and then adopted more widely within the NHS professional groups.

In the modern NHS, professions are rightly expected to work collaboratively for the benefit of the patient, but Hall (2005) described that the way different professional groups are educated and their histories can lead to differences in culture, language and the way problems are tackled. This has the potential to create professional silos, rather than support an interprofessional team. Hall (2005) gives examples of physicians being educated to lead, to take charge and to take responsibility for clinical decisions, at the same time the tradition of this leadership sets an expectation amongst other professionals that the physician will lead. Equally, the physician is likely to emphasise the scientific values in the form of blood test results, scans, for example, as weighty reasons for a particular clinical decision, whereas nurses may be more likely to emphasise how the patient is coping with their illness on a day-to-day basis. In some areas of complex need, there will be numerous individuals from different professional backgrounds each with their own set of expertise and their own views on what is to be valued. Agreement on treatment and on care planning can be influenced by these different professional values. Open communication and interprofessional trust and respect will enable better sharing and agreement about clinical decisions and effective teamwork can lead to more creative ways of working and more successful outcomes. The importance of the patient having a collaborative role in care decisions can sometimes seem to be at odds with the notion of the professional expert. While all health professionals value quality of life, an individual patient may see their life in a different way to the health professionals.

However, despite the desire for collaboration, Broukhim et al. (2019) argue that team work between health care professionals inevitably involves conflict. Their research highlighted a common cause of conflict between nursing and medical professionals with issues of power and hierarchy having the potential to override their shared values in relation to patient care. In their review, Paradis and Whitehead (2015) identify power and conflict as central elements in working together in interprofessional teams, linking these to both institutional and structural factors at work in large health organisations. Thus, the way in which an organisation is structured can affect the way in which power and hierarchy are held, and can impact the values which the professionals aspire to. A Canadian study by Brown et al. (2011) explored interprofessional conflict and found that different professionals were not always clear about the roles of the individual members of the interprofessional team and their scope of practice. Overlap may occur between areas of expertise which can cause conflict. The question of accountability also caused conflict, was each member of the team accountable, or did the physician have overall accountability? Hall (2005) also identified that because different health professionals are largely educated separately from each other, there can be a lack of understanding of the values held by other professions and potential mistrust within an interprofessional team. Interprofessional problem solving is not easy if the professional groups do not understand the values driving their thinking. Hall recommends open communication of reasoning and values between professionals to support professional respect and improved teamwork.

Even within a professional group there can be different values to consider. For example, Vatne and Fagermoen (2007, p. 41) considered the challenges for mental health nurses as to whether they should aim to 'correct' the behaviour of their clients, focusing on the external, or whether instead they should work from their values of compassion and the importance of patient integrity to enable their clients to change themselves from within. A similar challenge is considered by Robinson et al. (2007), should professionals always emphasise patient-centred care, even when the client has severe dementia? Their article explores the sort of everyday considerations which health professionals have to make, in this case the value placed on the safety of the client, and the prevention of harm to client and others, against the value of client independence and autonomy. An example from midwifery is provided by Fontein-Kulpers et al. (2018), in this case the dilemma midwives face when their values for high quality care, for which they are accountable and must meet both professional standards and standards of interprofessional care, do not match what the pregnant woman wants. These are everyday challenges for health care professionals and highlight the importance of professional judgement. When considering the imposition of changes, the professional judgement of the health care professional, and the flexibility to decide which values take precedence in different situations, must not be undermined.

Policy and the structure of the NHS

In the early days of the NHS, government ministers tended to take a hands-off approach and let administrators and managers run the service. This position has not continued. In the current situation, government ministers intervene and political interference is commonplace, especially in England. The intensity of political meddling has led many voices to plead for politics to be taken out of health care. However, health care is a political issue globally, even in countries where it is privatised, leading the Kings Fund to state

> It is pretty much impossible to completely 'depoliticise' the NHS, although it may be possible – and at times has been in the past even in England – to have ministers less involved in the day-to-day decisions about how the service operates.
>
> *(Timmins, 2018, p. 13)*

The NHS in the UK was established with the principle of providing free health care to the population irrespective of the ability to pay. This principle is upheld to the present day. However, since its inception much has changed in the country. There is now a larger and growing population needing health care, an increasing elderly population, new technology, trends in new diseases and increased costs of providing health care (Anandaciva et al., 2017). Alongside these challenges, the NHS is the largest employer in Europe consisting of a range of clinical, professional, technical, support and other staff.

The culture and values of the health service are clearly intertwined with politics, and changes in government policy have led to changes in the structure of the NHS and changed ways of working. Such changes have often been imposed on the health professionals working in the system, without acknowledging or measuring the impact of the changes. This section provides more detail to explain how such a complex system of health care provision has arisen and the implications for the professionals working within it.

At the heart of the relentless changes to healthcare in the UK is the question of how it should be financed and managed and these issues are based on political ideologies. Subsequent governments have sought to impose change as methods of addressing the spiralling cost of health care and its perceived inefficiencies and ineffectiveness. Each new government states that they have the answers to address the ills of the NHS. Often the changes are sold on the grounds of providing high quality, efficient and effective health care to the population, things that are of course wanted and needed.

The two main political parties in the UK have taken different approaches and view the challenges of the NHS in different ways. On the one hand, the Conservatives view inefficiencies as the fundamental issue, while the Labour party sees the main issue to be underfunding. While, typically, it has been the two main political parties imposing their ideological positions on the NHS, in 2010, a coalition government came into power and thus a new set of policies were instituted. This created a period of the greatest upheaval in the history of the NHS leading Ham et al. (2015, p. 4) to state:

> Historians will not be kind in their assessment of the coalition government's record on NHS reform. The first half of the 2010–15 parliament was taken up with debate on the Health and Social Care Bill, the biggest and most far-reaching legislation in the history of the NHS – designed (largely by the Conservative party in opposition) to extend the role of competition within the NHS and devolve decision-making.

Such a major change has taken its toll on staff health and wellbeing. We now consider some of the changes imposed by policies since the inception of the NHS.

1948–1983

Nicholas Timmins 2018 Report 'The World's Biggest Quango: The First Five Years of NHS England', while emphasising the huge and unintended changes occurring in NHS England during the first 5 years of its operation, also provides a political perspective on the NHS from its inception to the present day. In his report, he relays the involvement of successive governments in the NHS, emphasising the implementation of the Coalition government's policies and concluding that it is a challenge to separate healthcare policy from its implementation.

He discusses how, at the creation of the NHS in 1948 right up to the 1980s, the government's role was that of an administrator, although in the 1970s re-organisation there was an attempt by the government of the day to introduce 'command and control' (Timmins, 2018, p. 16). He indicates that from 1948 right up until 1974 there was no political intent by governments of the day. It was set up as a service which needed to be administered not managed. At the creation of the NHS, Regional Boards were set up to run nationalised hospitals. Ministers appointed the Boards but the Boards were independent of the Department of Health (DoH). Similarly, GPs were independent practitioners. In 1962, when major changes were proposed to the NHS by the then Minister, including building large numbers of hospitals, the role of the DoH remained an advisory one to the Regional Hospital Boards.

However, the re-organisation of 1974 was a turning point and the first attempt at government control over the NHS. Thus, services that were within the domain of local government were transferred into the NHS. These included public health, district nursing and health visiting, midwifery, school services and the ambulance service. Health authorities were created, replacing the Regional Boards, and with a wider brief. Suddenly, responsibility for the health of their local population was within their remit, not just responsibility for hospitals. Once again, ministers were involved in very senior appointments, but the health authorities were not part of the DoH. It could be argued that, in these first 35 years of the NHS, the structures were clear and understood nationally by both the staff of the NHS and by the population who sought to make use of it. The NHS existed to provide a universal health service but it was not run as a business and not run for profit. While it could be described as paternalistic (Klein, 2008), the service worked on professional capability and trust, and provision was based on health need. It had, however, become much more bureaucratic as a result of the 1974 changes.

1983–1987

It was the Griffiths' Report in 1983 that created major change to how the NHS would run. While up to this period the NHS was managed by administrators, this role was now to be undertaken by general managers. A complicated structure emerged in an attempt to show that the government in power would not meddle in the NHS, but reality proved otherwise. The new structure included a Management Board, chaired by a general manager (who was appointed by the Secretary of State) to manage the whole of the NHS, but accountable to the Supervisory Board which in turn was chaired by the Secretary of State.

So, it would be the Management Board, not politicians, managing the NHS. The idea was that the management of the NHS would not involve the government of the day. Its role was distinct and different, strategic not management, setting objectives but not making decisions about how these objectives should be achieved. Timmins (2018) suggests, however, that it was difficult to keep policy and operational aspects separate then and is even more so now. The challenge for ministers was that they considered both Parliament and the media held them accountable for performance of the NHS.

1987–1997

A review of the NHS under a Conservative government led by Margaret Thatcher created the purchaser/provider split, though many saw this as the creation of the 'internal market' which was heralded by ministers as 'decentralisation' (Timmins, 2018, p. 23). Timmins (2018) suggests that although it was referred to as the internal market, this was not the case. Health authorities and GPs became commissioners of services, with the job of purchasing care from the NHS, the private or the voluntary sector who were the providers of care. GPs now held budgets to purchase the care that their patients required.

The underpinning principle was that NHS hospitals would become independent, increasing competition amongst NHS Trusts and giving the autonomy to manage their Trusts as they wished, without interference from the government of the day. In effect each of the Trusts were to be businesses akin to GP practices, though much larger businesses. It was claimed that in practice 'money would follow the patient' (Timmins, 2018, p. 22) through competition successful businesses would increase their income and, in order to compete in the market, Trusts would increase efficiency and quality.

With ongoing financial challenges, the government found itself in a situation where it had to renege on these principles. The NHS was not allowed to keep any profits made creating tensions about the role of politics in the NHS. A separation of politics from the NHS was attempted by Kenneth Clarke, the Secretary of State for Health during this period. He created a 'policy board' which was a new version of the 'supervisory board' and a non-statutory arrangement turned the Management Board into an Executive within the DoH.

According to one of the interviewees in Timmins (2018) Report, William Waldegrave, this threw up the same issues as before, management were not free to manage, policymakers wanted more direct input into decisions about how objectives should be met. Decentralisation proved to be short-lived as financial controls gained the upper hand. While hospitals and GPs had some level of autonomy, essentially it was the government who was the driver of the market.

With this policy came criticisms of government interference, the power of commissioners, and increased spending on management. Further changes saw the 14 regional authorities reduced to 8, then 4, before they were abandoned. The NHS Executive was to oversee both policy and the decisions about how to implement that policy. The NHS had become a much more complex and more political organisation. Competition had been introduced, but political control had strengthened. The business model was quite distinct from its 1948 origins and the new structure was more cumbersome and less recognisable to its employees and the public.

1997–2010

A most dramatic change took place in 1997, by the then Labour government, when there was a major shift towards primary care. However, many would argue that the dramatic changes instituted under Tony Blair were more akin to Conservative ideologies rather than Labour. The policy change shift was towards primary care with a focus on prevention and public health. However, the internal market was created with purchasers and providers. PCTs were established to commission health care and hospitals became providers of health care. General Practice fundholding was de-established. Primary Care Groups were first created as commissioners, then turned into PCTs followed by mergers to reduce the numbers but the commissioning role remained. The internal market was created with a view to increasing productivity in the NHS, intending to address what the government felt was the reason for its problems. The Quality and Outcomes Framework of 2004, part of the new GP contract, reduced activity to measurable, priced units, enabling the use of software to codify the work of GPs. Not only did this increase the administrative load, its focus was away from the human side of medicine (Bunting, 2020).

The justification for the policy changes was on the grounds of giving patients choice and the need for competition and thus a range of services were commissioned from the independent sector. These included surgical treatment centres, and the private sector was further commissioned to treat NHS patients on waiting lists. The government also sought to open up the market in General Practice by encouraging for-profit companies to compete with GPs to deliver care.

Regional health authorities, which were disbanded, were now recreated into 28 health authorities, then merged again to reduce the numbers to 10. Large Foundation Hospitals and independent treatment centres were formed. The internal market proved a challenge. Although PCTs were commissioners, their lack of power meant that hospitals ate up the vast majority of the NHS funding (Miller *et al.*, 2012). What then followed was huge financial deficit and efforts to re-balance the books. Hospitals were reconfigured, jobs were frozen and some were cut. Added to this problem, it emerged that the costs for delivering the Information Technology (IT) plans were escalating with the delivery target unmet. Meanwhile an ongoing outbreak of methicillin resistant *Staphylococcus aureus* and increasing numbers of infections with *Clostridium difficile* were causing concern that the NHS was collapsing (Day, 2007).

Once again, the NHS had changed, with increased complexity in its structure, a focus on metrics and targets, and less easily understood either by those working within it or by those trying to make use of it.

2010–2020

A Conservative and Liberal Democrat Coalition UK Government was formed in 2010, leading to publication of numerous health care policies including Equity and Excellence, Liberating the NHS (DoH, 2010), Health and Social Care Act (2012), NHS Five Year Forward View (2014), and NHS Long Term Plan (2019). While the 1997 reforms could be viewed as a dramatic shift towards primary care and an introduction of the internal market, the coalition government's NHS policies could be viewed as the largest single change to the NHS structure in its history and a shift in the balance of power with far reaching changes, in particular the role of the economic regulator and the promotion of competition. Choice and competition were stated to be at the heart of the Health and Social Care Act, 2012. One aspect that caused much anxiety was that the government policy at the time allowed NHS services to be delivered by private providers (Timmins, 2018). The notion of social enterprises was introduced and much encouraged and an economic regulator was introduced, its function to encourage competition, deal with pricing and aim to ensure services continued (Ham *et al.*, 2015). The stated aim of these new policies was to create an independent NHS to run a 'quasi-market' and to remove the politics from it. NHS England was established as a statutory independent board with this role, instead it has been labelled as 'the World's biggest quango' (Timmins, 2018, p. 10). These policies caused some of the most challenging changes to the NHS.

The stated idea of the new healthcare policy was to keep politics out of the NHS. Thus, the NHS Commissioning Board was independent (NHS England)

and it was to be a 'lean and expert organisation, free from day-to-day political interference' (DoH, 2010, p. 30). Rather than being managed by the Commissioning Board, power was to be given to the front-line clinicians and patients. At the time of these proposals, many concerns were raised about the magnitude of the change and the potential outcome especially when the country was facing financial demands. According to Dixon and Ham (2010), justification for the change had not been given. Nevertheless, policy implementation continued.

Thus, the policies of the Labour government were overturned. The commissioning of health care was now to be undertaken by GPs and an independent NHS Commissioning Board was to take financial responsibility and a supervision role over GPs in their new capacity as commissioners. Both the strategic health authorities (SHAs) and PCTs were de-established. CCGs led by clinicians replaced PCTs. The structures put in place by the previous government were dissolved. This included the NHS Executive; the 152 PCTs which previously commissioned services; and the 10 SHAs which lay above PCTs. The focus on primary care has continued with the stated aim of addressing inequalities and prevention (NHS Long Term Plan, NHS, 2019).

A new outcomes framework for holding the NHS Commissioning Board to account was formed. Public health, which was part of the NHS, was moved to local authorities. All services such as health visiting, school nursing and other public health services now therefore moved to local authorities, so that individuals found themselves with new managers, new contracts and a great deal of confusion amongst health professionals and the general public. Services, buildings and people were changing hands, at times over and over again.

All Trusts became NHS Foundation Trusts. While this began slowly, the pace soon increased with further configuration and re-configuration of failed organisations. Organisations merged services, staff and departments to create even bigger Trusts. At the same time, there was re-deployment of staff, redundancies, new ways of working, redesign of services and more change to merge Trusts due to financial pressures. The general public, as recipients of health services, found hospital titles, service arrangements, individual staff roles and other areas changing frequently, with a lack of continuity in their experience. Competition grew and private providers provided a range of services for the NHS.

The NHS Five Year Forward View policy was introduced in 2014 with a new vision for the NHS underpinned by seven models of care: multispecialty community providers; primary and acute care systems; urgent and emergency care networks; acute care collaborations; specialised care; modern maternity services; and enhanced health in care homes. However, more changes are afoot.

Recent developments, 2021

The current pandemic (writing in April 2021) has put unprecedented demands on the NHS over the last year. Change has been a key feature within all settings. New technologies have been introduced leading to new ways of working. For example, the Nightingale hospital was created in 10 days, some GPs and consultants have made use of technology to manage appointments with patients, and staff have shown that they can adapt and adopt new ways of working. Many staff have had to be re-trained to take on roles caring for patients with Covid 19, senior clinicians and hospital consultants have been re-deployed to manage Covid and non-Covid settings as the situation has continued to change. The emotional toll has been high and continues to be so with many staff openly discussing the emotional impact of the pandemic and the change it has brought to their role. Unfortunately, in some areas, the response to change has been less creative, with some GP practices reducing the use of technology, removing on line bookings and consultations with patients being held by telephone rather than by some means which would enable the GP to see the patient, albeit through a computer screen. One result of the pandemic is longer waiting lists for patients, not just for routine visits but also for potentially life changing conditions. Some 6 million fewer referrals for tests and treatment were made by GPs over the last year during the pandemic. The pandemic has also highlighted the difference in values between the private sector and the NHS, illustrated by the awards of contracts to private organisations which have not had the experience or resources to deliver on promises. The latest proposals by government for further changes to NHS England have been identified in Chapter 1, suggesting that learning has not taken place at this level about the complexity of change nor about effective change management.

The general public and the NHS

Having explored some of the impacts of NHS changes on the staff who work within it in Chapter 1, we now turn briefly to the views of the people who use the NHS, the general public.

With so many changes in its history, and in the year of the 70th anniversary of the establishment of the NHS, Burkitt et al. (2018) considered the views of the British public. Their research demonstrated the pride which British people have in the NHS. The British public are pleased to have an NHS and speak highly of it. The authors are clear to point out, however, that public satisfaction with the management of the NHS has flagged, with dissatisfaction for some about their own experiences of the service. The public are well aware of the pressures which the NHS is under, both financial challenges and increased demand, but many consider the NHS as a 'bit of a mess' (Burkitt et al., 2018, p. 12) that could be better managed, both locally and nationally, and that there could be less waste. The use of agency staff, the large number of managers, use of the private sector and lack of re-use of consumables were some of the areas where participants in the study considered there was considerable and unnecessary waste. Many questioned the efficiency of the service. There was criticism about the increasing difficulty of accessing GPs when needed, and additional criticism about the poor organisation of the NHS, for example with last minute cancellations of services and appointments, poor IT systems, and poor communication. The system is complex to understand and at times challenging to access.

The changes to the NHS over time mean that there is now more emphasis within the NHS on the individual's responsibility for their health, a less paternalistic stance than there once was. The study confirmed that individuals believed they should indeed take responsibility for their own health but that the NHS should provide better support and information to those who want to make healthier changes to their lives and better guidance on how to use the services that are available.

Summary

We sought to explore and discuss the complexities in the NHS. With a large and complicated organisation such as the NHS, with many individual acute Trusts, large numbers of general practices in primary care, specialist services such as mental health, child, learning disability, together with a tranche of different professional disciplines, it is a challenge to create a common culture. Patients may be surprised to find there is no common culture. However, policy changes by successive governments have influenced a change in culture at the organisational level towards a culture of competition, targets, outcomes and value for money. This is in direct contrast to the culture of the members of the workforce who might see their job as a calling embedded by a culture of caring, compassion, people first, collaboration and harmony.

The wide range of professionals in the NHS are accountable to a variety of professional and regulatory bodies. Their values may not only be somewhat different across professions but also at odds with the values of the executives, managers and leaders of their organisation. The potential for conflict is high especially during change management where leaders might impose change from the top with little regard for the culture and values of the professional workforce who are already enduring high levels of emotional labour.

With the differing cultures and values in healthcare, it is unrealistic to expect a common culture for all. Leaders of change need to respect and harness the varying cultures and values of the different professional disciplines, technical and support staff, and working groups, instead of working against these. Despite the statements of values by the NHS in the different countries of the UK, staff at the frontline, and the patients themselves, do not always see these values evident in the way the system works. Staff face challenges to maintain their own professional values, which at times are at odds with the way the organisation functions.

From its early years with a clear structure which was understood by staff and patients alike, we have described how the NHS has become a political football, with numerous changes in policy over successive governments. There have been extensive changes, especially in NHS England. The policy changes have had national and local impact and have created a very large and sometimes disjointed and fragmented service which is not well understood by those who work in it or by those who require its services. Disappointingly, there is little work to suggest that these incessant changes have contributed any positive benefit to the health of the nation. They have been costly financially and have also been costly in terms of staff wellbeing and patient satisfaction, with both showing a decline in recent years.

Innovation, service improvement and development should continue to be a part of health care but leaders of change must consider the complexity of healthcare in change management and always put their most precious resources, that is people, at the centre of change. Later in the book, we demonstrate that through the assessment of emotional and cognitive readiness for change, change leaders will get to hear the voices of the workforce and can put in place strategies to harmonise the differing cultures and values towards a unified culture of quality improvement in healthcare informed by professionals and their clinical experience.

References

Anandaciva, S., Jabbal, J., Maguire, D. & Chijoko, L., 2017. *Quarterly Monitoring Report 24*. Kings' Fund. Available at: kingsfund.org.uk

Broukhim, M., Yuen, F., McDermott, H., Miller, K., Merrill, L., Kennedy, R., & Wilkes, M., 2019. 'Interprofessional conflict and conflict management in an educational setting'. *Medical Teacher*, 41(4): 408–416.

Brown, J., Lewis, L., Ellis, K., Stewart, M, Freeman, R.T., & Kasperski, M.J., 2011. 'Conflict on interprofessional primary health care teams: Can it be resolved?'. *Journal of Interprofessional Care*, 25(1): 4–10.

Bunting, M., 2020. *Labours of Love*. London: Granta Publications.

Burkitt, R., Duxbury, K., Evans, H., Ewbank, L., Gregory, F., Hall, S., Wellings, D., & Denzel, L., 2018. *The Public and the NHS: What's the Deal?* London: Kings Fund.

Campbell, D., 2021. 'Non-NHS healthcare providers given £96bn in a decade, says Labour, 3.5.2021'. *The Guardian*.

Campbell, H., 2008. '"Nothing about me, without me": NHS values past and future in Northern Ireland'. In Greer, S.L., & Rowland, D. (eds.), *Devolving Policy, Diverging Values? The Values of the United Kingdom's National Health Services*. Research Report. London: The Nuffield Trust. Available at: www.nuffieldtrust.org.uk/research/devolving-policy-diverging-values

Carroll, J.S., & Quijada, M.A., 2003. 'Redirecting traditional professional values to support safety: Changing organisational culture in health care'. *Qual Saf Health Care*, 13(Supplement II): ii16–ii21.

Davies, H., & Mannion, R., 2013. 'Will prescriptions for cultural change improve the NHS?'. *BMJ*, 346: 1–4. https://doi.org/10.1136/bmj.f1305

Day, M., 2007. 'C. difficile infections rise: But MRSA rates drop'. *BMJ*, 334: 924.

Dayan, M., & Edwards, N., 2017. *Learning from Scotland's NHS*. London: Nuffield Trust. Available at: www.nuffieldtrust.org.uk/files/2017-07/learning-from-scotland-s-nhs-final.pdf

Dayan, M., & Heenan, D., 2019. *Change or Collapse. Lessons from the Drive to Reform Health and Social Care in Northern Ireland*. London: Nuffield Trust. Available at: www.nuffieldtrust.org.uk/files/2019-07/nuffield-trust-change-or-collapse-web-final.pdf

Department of Health, 2010. *Equity and Excellence: Liberating the NHS*. London: The Stationery Office. Available at: https://assets.publishing.service.gov.uk/government/uploads/system/uploads/attachment_data/file/213823/dh_117794.pdf

Department of Health, 2012. *Compassion in Practice*. London: DoH. Available at: https://www.england.nhs.uk/wp-content/uploads/2012/12/compassion-in-practice.pdf (england.nhs.uk)

Dixon, A., & Ham, C., 2010. *'Liberating the NHS': The Right Prescription in a Cold Climate*. London: The King's Fund. Available at: https://www.kingsfund.org.uk/sites/default/files/Liberating%20the%20NHS%20-%20The%20right%20prescription%20in%20a%20cold%20climate1.pdf (kingsfund.org.uk)

Edwards, N., & Buckingham, H., 2020. *Strategic Health Authorities and Regions: Lessons from History*. Research Report. London: Nuffield Trust.

Fontein-Kulpers, Y., den Harthog van Veen, H., Klop, L., & Zondag, L., 2018. 'Conflicting values experienced by Dutch midwives: Dilemmas of loyalty, responsibility and selfhood'. *Clinical Research in Obstetrics and Gynaecology*, 1(1): 1–12. Available at: hogeschoolrotterdam.nl

Francis, R., 2013. *Report of the Mid Staffordshire NHS Foundation Trust Public Inquiry*. London: The Stationery Office.

General Medical Council, 2013. *Good Medical Practice*. London: GMC. Available at: www.gmc-uk.org/ethical-guidance/ethical-guidance-for-doctors/good-medical-practice

Greer, S.L., & Rowland, D. (eds.), 2008. *Devolving Policy, Diverging Values? The Values of the United Kingdom's National Health Services*. Research Report. London: The Nuffield Trust. Available at: www.nuffieldtrust.org.uk/research/devolving-policy-diverging-values

Hall, P., 2005. 'Interprofessional teamwork: Professional cultures as barriers'. *Journal of Interprofessional Care*, Supplement 1: 188–196.

Ham, C., 2014. *Reforming the NHS from Within: Beyond Hierarchy, Inspection and Markets*. London: King's Fund.

Ham, C., Baird, B., Gregory, S., Jabbal, J., & Alderwick, H., 2015. *The NHS Under the Coalition Government. Part One: NHS Reform*. London: King's Fund.

Health and Care Professions Council, 2016. *Standards of Conduct, Performance and Ethics*. London: HCPC. Available at: www.hcpc-uk.org/standards/standards-of-conduct-performance-and-ethics/

Health and Social Care Act, 2012. *UK Government Archives*. Available at: https://www.legislation.gov.uk/ukpga/2012/7/contents/enacted

Kerr, D., & Feeley, D., 2008. 'Collectivism and collaboration in NHS Scotland'. In Greer, S.L., & Rowland, D. (eds.), *Devolving Policy, Diverging Values? The Values of the United Kingdom's National Health Services*. Research Report. London: The Nuffield Trust. Available at: www.nuffieldtrust.org.uk/research/devolving-policy-diverging-values

The Kings Fund, 2017. *How Does the NHS in England Work? An Alternative Guide*. London: The Kings Fund. Available at: www.kingsfund.org.uk/audio-video/how-does-nhs-in-england-work. Last accessed 28.12.2020.

Klein, R. 2008. 'Values talk in the (English) NHS'. In Greer, S.L., & Rowland, D. (eds.), *Devolving Policy, Diverging Values? The Values of the United Kingdom's National Health Services*. Research Report. London: The Nuffield Trust. Available at: www.nuffieldtrust.org.uk/research/devolving-policy-diverging-values

Longley, M., 2015. 'Prudent progress in the Welsh NHS'. *Nuffield Trust Comment*, 29 July 2015. Blog post. Available at: www.nuffieldtrust.org.uk/news-item/prudent-progress-in-the-welsh-nhs

Mannion, R., Harrison, S., Jacobs, R., Konteh, F., Walshe, K., & Davies, H., 2009. 'From cultural cohesion to rules and competition: The trajectory of senior management culture in English NHS hospitals, 2001–2008'. *Journal of the Royal Society of Medicine*, 102(8): 332–336.

Marshall, M.N., Mannion, R., Nelson, E., & Davies, H.T.O., 2003. 'Managing change in the culture of general practice: Qualitative case studies in primary care trusts'. *BMJ*, 327: 599–602.

Michael, P., & Tanner, D., 2008. 'Values vs policy in NHS Wales'. In Greer, S.L., & Rowland, D. (eds.), *Devolving Policy, Diverging Values? The Values of the United Kingdom's National Health Services*. Research Report. London: The Nuffield Trust. Available at: www.nuffieldtrust.org.uk/research/devolving-policy-diverging-values

Miller, R., Peckham, S., Checkland, K., Coleman, A., McDermott, I., Harrison, S., & Segar, J., 2012. *Clinical Engagement in Primary Care-led Commissioning: A Review of the Evidence*. Technical Report. Policy Research Unit in Commissioning and the Healthcare System. London: London School of Hygiene and Tropical Medicine PRU-Comm. Available at: https://researchonline.lshtm.ac.uk/id/eprint/4648265/1/Clinical%20engagement%20in%20primary%20care_VoR.pdf (core.ac.uk)

Morgan, P., & Ogbonna, E., 2008. 'Subcultural dynamics in transformation: A multi-perspective study of healthcare professionals'. *Human Relations*, 6(1): 39–65.

NHS, 2019. *NHS Long Term Plan*. Available at: https://www.longtermplan.nhs.uk/

NHS Five Year Forward View, 2014. *NHS England*. Available at: https://www.england.nhs.uk/five-year-forward-view/

The NHS Constitution for England, 2021. Available at: www.gov.uk

NHS Scotland, 2013. *Everyone Matters: 2020 Workforce Vision*. The Scottish Government. Available at: www.gov.scot

Nursing and Midwifery Council, 2015. *The Code: Professional Standards of Practice and Behaviour for Nurses, Midwives and Nursing Associates*. London: NMC.

Nursing and Midwifery Council, 2017. *Joint Statement from the Chief Executives of Statutory Regulators of Health and Care Professionals 08.08.2017*. Available at: nmc.org.uk

Paradis, E., & Whitehead, C.R., 2015. 'Louder than words: Power and conflict in interprofessional education articles, 1954–2013'. *Medical Education*, 49(4): 399–407.

Robinson, L., Hutchings, D., Corner, L., Finch, T., Hughes, J., Brittain, K., & Bond, J., 2007. 'Balancing rights and risks: Conflicting perspectives in the management of wandering in dementia'. *Health, Risk & Society*, 9(4): 389–406.

Scott, T., Mannion, R., Marshall, M., & Davies, H., 2003. 'Does organisational culture influence health care performance? A review of the evidence'. *Journal of Health Services Research & Policy*, 8(2): 105–117.

Sturgeon, D., 2014. 'The business of the NHS: The rise and rise of consumer culture and commodification in the provision of healthcare services'. *Critical Social Policy*, 34(3): 405–416.

Timmins, N., 2018. *The World's Biggest Quango: The First Five Years of NHS England*. London: Institute for Government & The Kings Fund. Available at: worlds_biggest_quango_ifg_may2017.pdf (kingsfund.org.uk)

Vatne, S., & Fagermoen, M.S., 2007. 'To correct and to acknowledge: Two simultaneous and conflicting perspectives of limit-setting in mental health nursing'. *Journal of Psychiatric and Mental Health Nursing*, 14(1): 41–48.

Vincent, C., 2010. *Patient Safety* (2nd ed.). Chichester, UK: Wiley Blackwell BMJ Books.

Willis, D.W., Saul, J., Bevan, H., Scheirer, M.A., Best, A., Greenhalgh, T., Mannion, R., Cornelissen, E., Howland, D., Jenkins, E., & Bitz, J., 2016. 'Sustaining organizational culture change in health systems'. *Journal of Health Organization and Management*, 30(1): 2–30.

3
A CRITIQUE OF CHANGE MANAGEMENT THEORIES AND APPROACHES

Introduction

The plethora of models, approaches, theories and improvement tools for managing change is overwhelming. In 2001, the NHS undertook a global review of change approaches and produced a report, available for use by NHS staff. Unfortunately, no guidance was given on which might be the most effective approach amongst the array of ideas. Successive governments continue to give enormous resources towards managing change with scant reference to the success or failure of current change approaches. National change agencies have been established and disbanded only to reemerge. External consultancies and companies continue to be commissioned to manage change. However, the failure rate for change initiatives can be up to 70% (Sackman et al., 2009; Burnes & Jackson, 2011; Burnes, 2017). There are individual reports of change success in the UK health sector, however, in general, there have not been consistent or sustainable change successes.

The tranche of Change Management Models, approaches and tools are underpinned by differing philosophies, values and beliefs. Some of these conflict with each other, while others do not have any theoretical foundation (Burnes, 2014, 2017). There is currently no unified view on how healthcare change should be managed, nor is there clear evidence of which approaches, models and tools are used, their rate of success or failure in individual Trusts, regionally or nationally. There is a lack of health care-based approaches to assist change and the gap in the literature and research for health care change is a potential challenge. We are bombarded with information on change management from the NHS Improvement website and from diverse sources issuing edicts and giving advice. However, the principal challenge remains, the vast majority of these Change Management Models, approaches and tools tend to focus on changing people's thinking only, often treating people as machines and not considering the entirety of human nature. The

DOI: 10.4324/9781003128397-3

language and tone of these approaches, models and tools is often technical, almost robotic in persuading people to accept and work with change. With evidence pointing to the failure of current change management approaches in health care, we argue that new thinking is required. People do not function with either cognition or emotion but with both. Thus, cognitive and emotional readiness for change is potentially the key to successful change management.

We focus our discussion on the popular approaches in the literature. This chapter begins the exploration of a number of planned, emergent and improvement approaches to change management and endeavours to identify the strengths and perceived weaknesses of such approaches. With quality improvement high on the agenda for change we explore the popular methodologies in the literature. The limited research that has been undertaken by health care practitioners indicates a leaning towards the importance of human emotion in effective change management.

The planned approach to change

The planned and emergent approaches to change dominate the literature. The planned approach originated with Kurt Lewin (Lewin, 1951) and was the prevailing approach until the 1980s (Bamford & Forrester, 2003; Burnes, 2017). Many proponents of the planned approach view change as a transitional process moving from one state to the next, occurring in isolation and incrementally, and thus change needs to be pre-planned and directed from the top of the organisation downwards. Under the umbrella of the planned approach many other models have developed. However, Lewin's model is still a main driver in the planned approach to change (Burnes, 2014, 2017).

Lewin's theory

Kurt Lewin, a social scientist who worked to resolve social conflict first described what became a very widely used theory underpinning the management of change. Lewin (1951) first coined the term 'planned change' to distinguish from unintended or accidental changes which may happen to an organisation. The theory stresses the balance between forces which drive the planned change forward and forces which hold the change back. Cummings *et al.* (2016) emphasise the importance that Lewin gave to group dynamics, evident in Lewin's recommendation to undertake a force field analysis when planning change. Lewin stresses the significance of assessing the forces at work in an organisation, whether people, systems or procedures and policy, and their relative positive or negative strengths. He calls these 'driving forces' and 'restraining forces'. Visually mapping the forces, with arrows of different sizes and directions working for and against the change can give a picture from which to analyse the factors influencing change (a number of simple tools have been created to support this and are widely available on the internet). An idea of readiness for change can be understood here but no explicit statement about emotional or cognitive readiness is made. This element, encompassing group dynamics, is not always referred to when considering the use of Lewin's model for planned change. Cummings *et al.* (2016) note that much of the criticism of Lewin's model is of the simplicity of the three-stage process of change management (described in the following) which is often presented as the whole model, with linear steps. Common criticisms of Lewin's approach are addressed by Burnes (2004, 2017) who notes that the main critics appear not to have read most of Lewin's work, and instead consider only one element: the three-stage process. Cummings *et al.* (2016) present a powerful critique that the simplicity of the model did not originate from Lewin, but is to be found in secondary sources which have sought to simplify the process of change. The writers of the secondary sources from the 1980s, they argue, wanted a simpler process to fit with the technical approach to change which arose in this period. The importance of Lewin's work is emphasised by Rosenbaum *et al.* (2018) who herald the complexity and current relevance of Lewin's theories. As Burnes (2004) has shown, Lewin's planned approach to change comprised four elements: field theory and group dynamics provided a theoretical basis, aimed to detail the motivations for behaviours within groups, and action research and the three-stage process aimed to enable change. Burnes identifies the importance of considering all four elements of Lewin's work in this field, but highlights that they tend, now, to be treated as separate elements of his work.

The three-stage process proposed by Lewin when planning change includes:

- The unfreezing stage generates a feeling of the need for change and involves the employees in finding ways to change, and in selecting the best way to undertake the change. Best use is made of the driving forces and motivating the workforce.
- The moving stage redefines the current situation, plans are made and staff are involved in commenting on and trying out the change. Detailed further plans are made. A specialist or well-known powerful person may be used to support the change.
- Finally, the stage of freezing (often referred to as refreezing) reinforces the change and new working patterns, policies and procedures are put in place. The values implicit in the new change become embedded.

A number of authors have stated that Lewin's model can be useful in change management in the health service. For example, Suc *et al.* (2009) found Lewin's model, including the three-stage process, group dynamics and action research, very useful in making a change in health informatics in a university hospital in Germany; Tinkler *et al.* (2014) found the model useful in supporting improvements in compression bandaging technique for venous ulceration in a community nursing team in Northern Ireland. The model can also be used as an evaluative tool, for example Mehrolhassani and Emami (2013) made use of the three-stage element of the model to evaluate the implementation of an accounting system within the health sector in Iran.

The systematic review undertaken by Harrison et al. (2021) selected 38 studies in health care which had made use of change management methodology covering 10 different countries. Lewin's model, which was used in 11 of the studies, was second in popularity to Kotter's model (see in the following). Unfortunately, in the majority of cases, the model is confined to structural elements of the change, without much reference to group dynamics or action research. Two of the projects using Lewin's model were to improve nursing handover at the bedside (Bradley & Mott, 2014; Chaboyer et al., 2009). They used Lewin's model in a structural way, to frame the change, using the three-stage element of the model. In a further study of nursing handover, reference is made to the use of Lewin's three-stage model, but alongside Peplau's theory of interpersonal relations (Radtke, 2013). While not identifying the wider remit of Lewin's theory, clearly aspects of this (group dynamics) were part of the model used. Use of Lewin's model has not just been reported at local level, institutional level change has been reported with successful use of the three-stage element of Lewin's theory. Abd El-Shafy et al. (2019) reported success using the model to introduce a collaborative care model in a paediatric setting, reducing non-surgical trauma admissions. In a geriatric setting, a new model of care was introduced (Jacelon et al., 2011) making part use of Lewin's three-stage model, with a focus on the moving stage rather than the unfreezing and refreezing stages. It is not clear why the wider elements of Lewin's work were not used in these studies.

A Canadian study (Sutherland, 2013) of change in health care makes slightly wider use of Lewin's theory. The change took place in a large psychiatric unit and aimed to introduce new technology in the form of bar-coded medication. While focusing on Lewin's three-stage process, the importance of all stakeholders participating in the process of change is linked to reduction of emotional responses such as fear when change is to take place. Thus, there is an element of group dynamics implicit in this study.

Was Lewin still developing his theories about change when he died at the early age of 56? Cummings et al. (2016) imply this to be the case. His earlier theoretical work on group dynamics and action research demonstrates the depth of thought in development of these ideas; it would be reasonable to assume that Lewin had also considered the management of change, leading to the three-stage process, in considerable depth. The three-stage process has been elaborated by others during the time since Lewin's death in 1947, but remains very relevant in the 21st century. For example, in their consideration of Lewin's model in the constantly changing world of information technology, Sarayreh et al. (2013, p. 626) identified the importance of 'soft-side effects', or in other words, the people element of change. They describe Lewin as keen to embed democratic values into change management, and so resolve social conflict. They note the altruistic nature of Lewin but also the significant value Lewin gave to group behaviour, the human element of organisations. They challenge the criticism that Lewin's model is too simplistic for today's world, noting that having impact on the behaviour of people is an essential element in all organisations, whether to effect change or to maintain the status quo.

Kotter's model

A model of planned change which is very familiar to many in the health sector is Kotter's eight-stage model of planned change (Kotter, 1996). The model was one of those specifically promoted as enabling the seven success factors for change by the Health Foundation (Allcock *et al.*, 2015). Maclean and Vannet (2016) found that Kotter's theory of change was effective at changing practice at a national or regional level, using a top-down approach, although Baloh *et al.* (2017) found that the model is understudied in the health care sector. In the systematic review undertaken by Harrison *et al.* (2021) mentioned earlier, the most popular model used in the 38 selected studies was that of Kotter (half the studies made use of this model). However, Kotter's model was mainly used for changes at local level or within single units, or for quality improvement.

Kotter is considered to be one of the leading experts on transformational change and his ideas about the importance of taking time and energy to ensure the change works (i.e. seeing change through to full implementation) have been significant. His model also arises from the work of Lewin. The eight steps identified by Kotter are:

- Establish a sense of urgency
- Establish a team able to guide the change
- Develop a vision and strategy
- Communicate the vision widely
- Empower staff to act to achieve the vision
- Set short term achievable goals
- Keep the sense of urgency
- Make the changes last/endure

The model is a useful way of ensuring energy in change implementation, there is a 'drive' to the process, a sense of movement forward to implementation of the change. This could be seen as a way of engaging with the emotional needs of the staff to be involved as the change occurs, but it does not recognise the emotional impact of the change itself which is likely to occur at an individual level, especially with major change. The concept of readiness for change is somewhat overlooked by Kotter: the staff might be completely unreceptive to the change despite the establishment of a sense of urgency. Kotter himself acknowledges the challenges organisations face when trying to change people's behaviour (Kotter, 2002). Kotter's model also assumes that change will start at the top of the organisation and be imposed downwards. In his 2014 book, Kotter expounds the value of a good hierarchy for enabling the function of large organisations. He does, however, also acknowledge that hierarchical structures have limitations when it comes to effective change, tending to cause the formation of silos which limit both the ability to take risks and also the ability to enable creativity within the organisation. Instead, Kotter suggests the use of a network structure to enable 'many more people to become active agents of change' (Kotter, 2014, p. 14). Kotter is not here advocating elimination of a hierarchical structure, but rather a dual structure of both hierarchy and network, with the network element drawing from different parts of the organisation to work flexibly on different initiatives while drawing on the range of skills and experience available within the organisation. Notably, though, Kotter advocates such a network being initiated and sustained by top management (p. 21). His renewed presentation of the eight steps (Kotter, 2014, pp. 27–34) does not reference emotional or cognitive readiness but rather focuses on removal of barriers to change (p. 31). In this way, the individual employees involved and their experiences of change are not acknowledged.

Teixeira and Austin (2017) used Kotter's model as a structure for their research into a practice change in community pharmacy in Ontario, Canada. Their findings demonstrate the value of parts of Kotter's model when implementing change, but they also found real challenges when making changes in practice. The focus in this case had been a change in legislation and regulatory structure, in order to 'permit' change in practice. However, the change in legislation and regulation was not accompanied by processes to enable implementation of change at a local practice level. The complex nature of the health service and the need to communicate with such a large range of different people and professions, within different community practice settings, meant the message of change could be easily lost. Teixeira and Austin (2017) make an important statement, that individual experiences of practitioners may be divorced from the top-down decisions about change, so that enabling processes are not considered. Individual pharmacists had context specific needs which were not accounted for. They specifically note the 'stress and anxiety' (p. 204) experienced by community pharmacists but with no mechanism to identify and work with the causes of such stress. Thus, they found a deficiency in using Kotter's model, a lack of engagement with the individual emotional reactions to change creating a barrier to implementation of change. The complexity referred to by Teixeira and Austin (2017) is important and Chapter 2 of this book considers complexity and change in the health service.

At the beginning of this chapter, we mentioned the global review of change models undertaken in 2001 by the NHS, and the production of a report from this. It could be argued that at national level in the UK a similar problem occurred to that experienced by Teixeira and Austin (2017), permitting the change was not the same as enabling the change. The lack of guidance on how to select from the array of models and theories available meant that the research was not effectively transferred into practice.

Emotional connection is often overlooked when using Kotter's model to change practice. Despite Kotter (2002) writing about the 'see-feel' approach, the model itself lacks explicit reference to the range of emotional responses to change. Rather, the 'see-feel' element is about making the motivation for change more explicit through real examples rather than just stating the business case. In her article, Burden (2016) demonstrates the use of Kotter's model to bring about a reduction in surgical infection rates but despite arguing that Kotter emphasised the need to 'connect with . . . emotions' (p. 949), there is a lack of recognition of emotional response to change. Her use of terms such as 'stubbornness' (p. 954) suggest a lack of understanding of the emotional impact on individuals and an expectation that focusing on 'cognition' (p. 952) to help the staff understand and make the change will be enough. Although change may occur, without consideration of emotional as well as cognitive readiness it is likely that the change will not be sustained across the organisation. In his book, Kotter (2002) stresses that the see-feel approach is more effective than the analytical-think approach. This could be extended to understand how the employees 'see' and 'feel' the prospective change. Thus, Kotter's model has the potential to include the emotional element of change on individuals, but there is a lack of examples in the literature of this actually occurring.

Organisational development

Organisational development (OD) is a further structure to manage change which is based on the work of Kurt Lewin. Burnes and Cooke (2012) suggest that OD has been and continues to be the main way in which the western world goes about organisational change. However, the authors argue that the meaning of OD is understood differently by different people, with some considering it to have been a feature of the 1950s to the 1980s, before disappearing, while others consider that the early version was a form of Lewin's model, with the later version continuing to have a base in social constructionism but with a move away from Lewin. Their article provides the critical review of the development of OD which, they argue, is sadly lacking. Identifying OD as still relevant, they argue that it has lost some of the values and aims of its originators, and in its current form it is not able to do as it should, it is not suitable to enable change.

OD was originally rooted in Lewin's work. Lewin provided both a theoretical basis (field theory, group dynamics) as well as a means of enacting change in practice (action research, the three-stage model of change) and these components formed the fundamental elements from which OD developed. Lewin had shown how psychological theory could be used in practice to change behaviour based on his work on group dynamics. Lewin's work to address social conflict meant that the values underpinning changes within groups were based in democracy and participation (Burnes & Cooke, 2012) and early OD followed this with its three main elements: T-groups, action research and participative management. Lewin's workshops promoting participation within communities, to promote racial and cultural harmony, resulted in structures to promote change, known as T-groups, groups where individuals could consider their emotions, their feelings, their attitudes, receiving feedback to become more self-aware. This change in awareness of their own behaviour was considered as essential before the individual could start to change the behaviour of others. Burnes and Cooke (2012) saw this as very similar to the ideas of emotional intelligence. These T-groups were the starting point of the OD movement, but as the groups rapidly developed, without appropriate control or regulation, their effectiveness diminished. Action research initiatives then became more popular based on Lewin's ideas of group participation leading to common understanding of a situation.

By the 1970s and 1980s, a stronger top-down style of management was emerging and was perceived as the best way to deal with global competition and rapid response to the market. Organisations needed to be more effective and more profitable. With this was a move away from the fundamental values which Lewin had stressed, those of democracy, of resolution of social conflict, of group dynamics. The theoretical basis of OD in its early days was the inclusion of people through groups, and the promotion of self-awareness (including emotional self-awareness) necessary to support change. The move to focus on outcomes, rather than process, appears to have been a problem for OD as it looked to reconsider its theoretical and practical base.

Discussing the failure of large, corporate, international organisations to make effective change, Beer et al. (1990) describe the way careful planning, change in organisational structure and specific training have all failed to create the desired and planned-for change. Their research found that when one strategy to change failed, it was quickly replaced by another, which also failed to achieve the desired outcomes, with constant change having a negative impact on the organisation. They describe the need to change the hierarchical and managerially controlled change and instead enabling teams to generate ideas and strategies for change, working across organisational boundaries. This might suggest that Beer et al. (1990) are proposing a move away from planned change to ideas of emergent change. However, their 'six steps to effective change' (p. 161) suggests that although ideas might be generated within the workforce, a much more structured approach will then occur to enact the change.

The emergent approach to change

In contrast to the planned approach is the emergent approach, established with the view that change is unpredictable. In the modern 21st century world, global influences, changing systems and parameters and constant demand for improvements mean that the planned approach to change has significant limitations. These include failure rates for change initiatives of up to 70% (Sackman et al., 2009; Burnes & Jackson, 2011). It is argued by Burnes and Jackson (2011) that a key reason for such failures is that how the management see change, and how the rest of the staff see the same change, are not aligned, with a lack of concern by managers for the experiences of the workforce.

It is therefore unsurprising that a new approach to change emerged. Liebhart and Garcia-Lorenzo (2010, p. 216) use the terms 'unpredictable', 'unintentional' and 'iterative' to describe the emergent approach to change and Burnes (2017) emphasises the environmental shift which brings about emergent change, the continuous nature of the change as adaptation to a new environment occurs and the way in which the future way of working cannot be predicted. Protagonists of the emergent approach argue that organisations need to be in a state of readiness to navigate change (Bamford & Forrester, 2003) and therefore change should be driven from the bottom of the organisation. The emergent school spans from those who focus on analysing organisational processes, to those who prescribe how change should be managed, or to those who do not fall within the parameters of either (Pettigrew, 1985; Pettigrew *et al.*, 2001; Dawson, 2003; Kanter *et al.*, 1992; Luecke, 2003).

Whereas planned change is expected, and has a start and a finish point, emergent change occurs without deliberate planning, for example in response to a significant event which causes disequilibrium and a need for new ways of working. As it is unplanned, the change process is iterative, ways of working will emerge as things are tried out and adjusted within the new environment. With planned change there is a vision, an expected final outcome. This is not the case with emergent change where the outcome is often unable to be predicted. The events of 2020, with the need for a global response to a pandemic, have resulted in many examples of emergent change. Organisations have had to think differently to manage previously unknown situations and new ways of working (e.g. the potential of telephone and on-line consultations; the huge increase in remote working) and these are expected to change post-Covid 19 ways of working. The changes in working practices are not yet fixed (writing mid 2021) but will continue to develop in response to the new environment. Opportunities which had not been considered before the pandemic have now been forced upon organisations, but the final outcome is not yet a known one. This can of course create challenges for managers who find that they have to be receptive to changes which they themselves are not in control of.

Research by Liebhart and Garcia-Lorenzo (2010) found that while dealing with emergent change, there was still a wish for stability and a need to go back to known ways of coping in order to manage the emergent change. In reality, planned and emergent approaches to change will occur concurrently but planned approaches alone are insufficient in the rapidly changing and unpredictable world of the 21st century. The neatness of planned change is a concept rarely reflective of today's health care practice. Dawson (2003) criticises the sanitised stories often provided by large organisations which suggest that change is a series of successful steps in a linear process. He identifies organisational change as a much more complex set of competing factors, involving politics and power, which give rise to different stories of change. He argues for greater criticality in research about organisational change, a move away from a single narrative of the best way to effect change, to an understanding of the complexity of change, as different people and groups experience it, with their different values, aspirations and histories. He is critical of the idea that managers can be leaders of change by being driven by competition, noting that resistance to change, power struggles and the failure to change are real issues of significant importance. He also recognises that the rationale provided for change is often founded on only partial understanding of an issue, or a one-sided perspective provided by a powerful member of the team, so that the change ends up not addressing some of the other elements of the problem.

Writing in 2014, Antwi and Kale remarked that emergent change theory is still in development, and there is no 'principle theoretical foundation' (p. 7). Three theoretical models relate to the complexity of change. Hinings and Greenwood's model of change dynamics (Hinings & Greenwood, 1989; Greenwood & Hinings, 1996) presents the argument that the environment in which an organisation operates is constantly changing, and that neither the changes nor their consequences can be known beforehand (i.e. change is emergent). This is certainly true of the NHS. Because of this, organisations need to better understand the context in which the organisation operates and better understand their workforce. The model emphasises power dynamics which may operate during change between one part of the organisation and another, and that parts of the organisation may benefit from a change, while another part may not. Leadership is also emphasised in the model, but not in the sense of being able to gain ideas for change from the workforce, but rather to provide explanations of the agreed change and to engage staff to be enthusiastic about it. The model does not demonstrate understanding of the emotional reactions which staff may have to change. Rather, it is similar in this element to Kotter's model in supporting staff to be enthusiastic about change without understanding that other factors may be at play to make it difficult for staff to see the positive potential for change.

The complexity of change is also recognised in Kanter et al. (1992) who developed their Big Three model of organisational change. Focusing on the complexity of change, the model explains that the organisation is changing related to the external world, but also changing within itself, and that the people and groups within the organisation are also changing which may lead to internal power struggles. Kanter et al. (1992) call this *motion*. The change itself can take different *forms*, for example the identity of the organisation may shift, the way in which the different parts of the organisation work together may change and the power relationships within the organisation may shift. A third section of the model includes the different *roles* operating through change. For example, there may be someone who determines the overall strategy but who may not be part of the process of change itself. There will also be those whose role it is to ensure the change occurs, which Kanter et al. (1992) describe in terms of seeing through the process of a planned change. Finally, there is the role of those who will experience the change, described as recipients, but have been unable to input into what the change will be or how it will be enacted. There is considerable attention to detail, acknowledging the complexity of change and aimed at ensuring change is embedded. However, the model assumes top-down leadership, and does not appear to acknowledge the value of the workforce in being involved in planning for change.

Other theorists have pointed out the lack of relevant research of appropriate quality for change management. Pettigrew et al. (2001, p. 709) emphasise that much of the research into change management is of the 'what is' variety, whereas practitioners want to know 'how to'. They note that much of the work presented as best practice on management of change was based on research foundations that lacked rigour. These authors identify a need to consider the large number of contexts which operate within change, and particularly to consider not just what academic research might indicate, but also to consider how practitioners can make sense of change. They describe the need for organisations to consider the sequence of change, for example to enable the organisation to be best placed to enact future change.

One of the first theorists to consider major change in the NHS, Pettigrew has written widely about strategic change. Pettigrew et al. (1992, p. 27) remind us of the 'politically driven and top-down pressure for change' which was a feature of the 1980s NHS. At this time, greater and greater emphasis was being placed on the manager's ability to manage change. There was a considerable move in the public sector, an expectation of being more like the private sector in management. However, the trend was for change to be instigated and managed by an individual leader, with a range of 'fads and fashions, off-the-shelf solutions' (p. 27) rather than emphasis on well-researched evidence. The complexity of change, and the many different layers of activity and meaning in change, had been ignored. Pettigrew and Whipp (1993) saw that there can be competitive advantage to making changes and that these can give a sense of purpose, rather than just reacting to the changing external environment. They advocate that there must be consideration of the *context* of the change, both within and outside the organisation. Thus, the way in which the organisation is set up, the power dynamics and the staff and other resources should be considered in relation to the changing world external to the organisation. Their model also identifies the importance of leadership in providing a vision of the change and making it work, the *content*. Included here is the importance of understanding the change from the points of view of different people in the organisation. As a final element in change, the model considers *process*. This element is about ensuring there is understanding of the change, supporting the change through time, and working to reduce any resistance which may occur. Within this model, there is a clear emphasis on seeing the change through to full implementation, something which is often under emphasised in models of change.

Pettigrew and Whipp's model was developed from work with private organisations but was later used in the health care sector (Pettigrew *et al.*, 1992). Investigating eight district health authorities and the processes used for strategic change in service, Pettigrew *et al.* (1992) were able to draw out eight factors which suggested receptivity to change. For example, they found that policy was of a better standard and held together more effectively in organisations or groups with this receptivity and that organisational goals were clearer. In these more effective organisations, identified individuals led on the change, and individual workers found the organisation to be receptive and supportive in nature with good communication. Unlike models of planned change, there was no step-by-step approach to achieve such receptivity, instead, sensitivity to organisational context was emphasised. They note, however, that even where these factors were evident, 'there was no simple recipe of quick fix in managing complex change' (Pettigrew *et al.*, 1992, p. 31). This concept of receptivity suggests that some organisations are able to be in constant readiness for change, with the potential to exploit opportunities for emergent change. Pettigrew's contribution to our understanding of change includes recognition of change as a complex process which is far from linear and influenced by the culture of the organisation (Sminia, 2017). For effective change, it is important to work together with the various teams and individuals of an organisation to enable better insight into what problems need to be solved, or to identify novel solutions to those issues.

Pettigrew and Whipp's Content, Context and Process model of strategic change has been used as a theoretical framework to explore the features which enabled historic change to embed evidence in practice settings. Stetler *et al.* (2007) made the assumption that examples where evidence-based practice existed were at some point preceded by a successful change in practice. They researched the context (the why), content (the what) and the process (the how) of such change, thus demonstrating a useful tool for consideration of effectiveness of change.

Another theorist, described as 'a "great" in theory of change management' (Cooke, 2017, p. 1) is Bernard Burnes. His work is highly relevant and modern, and yet based in a similar ideology of social democracy and avoidance of social conflict to that of Kurt Lewin. We noted earlier in this chapter his insights into the way Kurt Lewin's model of change has been poorly applied. Burnes does not subscribe to a single 'best way' of managing change and is critical of the top-down approach which he sees as often failing to engage with solving the problem. He advocates the need to better understand situations through accepting that different stakeholders will experience a situation differently, only through understanding a situation will successful change be possible. Burnes argues that all change and the way change is carried out involves choices. For him, choosing an approach which is 'ethical and participative' (Cooke, 2017, p. 6) is fundamental to successful change and should be part of leadership (Burnes *et al.*, 2016). This suggests that leaders should be in tune with their workforce, able to listen to them and their ideas for change, and receptive to these ideas so that the workforce can influence the outcomes of change for the better. This involvement of the workforce in change is linked to better short- and long-term commitment from them as the change progresses (Burnes & Jackson, 2011). This style of participative leadership would enable readiness for change, as managers better understand the practitioners' experiences of change.

Emergent change theorists have provided not just ideas about what emergent change is, but also ideas about how leaders of change can adapt their ways of working to better include the workforce, and thus improve the success of change. It is clear to us that emergent change can have even greater impact on the emotions of individuals affected than planned change and the need for a model which includes recognition of emotional response to change is even more pressing.

Healthcare change and change models

Despite the large volumes of work about change management, Leybourne (2016) notes that much of the literature about change deals with change in for-profit organisations, and more work is required to support successful change in the public health care sector. This section briefly considers some of the guidance for change in the health sector in the UK and North America over the last two decades and whether these ideas fit within concepts of planned change, emergent change and emotional elements of change or whether they are unique to health care. Models such as the NHS Change Model devised by NHS England and others have yet to be evaluated and it is not clear whether they are being used effectively in the NHS to manage change. The Executive Summary for NHS England (2018a) states that health organisations that use a model for change are likely to have better results than those that do not, but they are unable to identify a specific model to recommend.

54 Critique of change management theories

The National Institute for Health and Clinical Excellence (NICE) is a UK wide organisation with its stated aim being to develop best practice through best evidence. Their remit is concerned with best clinical outcomes as well as cost effectiveness. In 2007, NICE produced a guide on how to change practice, with a subtitle of 'understand, identify and overcome barriers to change'. Within the document, people are identified as important components of any change in practice. NICE identifies people's 'priorities and commitments' and 'personal beliefs and attitudes' (NICE, 2007, p. 8) as possible barriers to change. The guidance is useful and includes emphasis on ensuring wide communication of both the need to change and how the change is being implemented. This acknowledges the importance of cognition in change, staff are provided with information which helps them to understand what is happening and why. However, in the section on how to overcome barriers to change, there is no acknowledgement of the need to engage with individuals or to consider that the change might have an emotional effect on them. An emphasis on readiness to change at an emotional level is not evident in this guide.

The NHS England (2018c) Change Model, developed first in 2010 and now in its fifth version, describes itself as a suitable framework for large-scale or small-scale change. It identifies itself as a framework rather than a methodology, and is not intended to be prescriptive. In this way it differs from the models of planned change discussed earlier in this chapter. A range of tools to support the framework are provided for use if required. There is no prescription for change management, instead there is an offer of elements to be considered and tools which could be useful. The framework emphasises the importance of people in change: 'improvement efforts work best if there is an explicit connection between the change and people's values' (p. 9) and recommends spending time on ensuring a 'shared purpose' (p. 9). This is to be applauded, and could be construed as developing readiness for change. However, the need to consider the way the team and organisation function, within a very complex network of health services and the people they are there to serve, and the often different or competing values held between different parts of the organisation, are not considered. Readiness for change could form a much larger component here. Under the section on motivate and mobilise, psychological factors are identified as an 'energy of change' (p. 21) which should be taken into account to harness the whole team. Thus, the NHS England Change Model does consider human nature. It includes taking into consideration motivation and other factors, but could go much further in being explicit about emotional and cognitive readiness for change.

'The Best Practice Change Management Guidelines' were released by the London Procurement Programme in 2010 (Phelan, 2010), as a means of managing the change to implementation of electronic rostering and/or software to manage bank staff. Early in the guidelines the significance of supporting staff within such a change is referred to. Phelan (2010) notes that even changes in technology require changes in staff working practices, and that 'The most common reason for an e-Rostering and/or staff bank solution failing to deliver the expected benefits is lack of acceptance and use by staff' (Phelan, 2010, p. 6). The mechanism used for implementing the change is a project management tool,

PRINCE2. Use of a project management approach implies making a planned change, with little scope for emergent change. The focus is on successful completion of the change through a series of steps. Exploring the approach for the way in which impact on staff is considered and mitigated, the approach appears mechanistic. For example, regional directors 'Could inform on expected reaction to change from workforce' (p. 7); a 'clinical specialist' (p. 8) could be part of the implementation team. The importance of having staff accept the change is stressed. During the design phase, there is emphasis on ensuring representation from different stakeholders and 'early engagement' (p. 9) with those affected by the change is suggested. Step 3 of the process, gaining commitment, includes a statement to 'assess readiness for change' (p. 11) but no detail is provided on how this might take place. Within the guidelines for implementation, there is no mention of the emotional response of staff or others and how this might be managed, and staff supported through what could be very significant change. There is no consideration that introduction of e-rostering could have an impact on patient experience and how this might be mitigated.

Discussing much bigger changes, NHS England (2018b) propose a model for Large Scale Change which includes the NHS Change Model. There is emphasis on the importance of 'commitment' (p. 33), 'shared goals, values and sense of purpose' (p. 33). This is described as a different approach to the 'compliance' (p. 33) typical in some organisations, which are driven by process and hierarchy. In this sense it is more people focused than some other models, but there is a lack of understanding of individual employees or patients' emotional responses to such large-scale change and no indication therefore of how these might be addressed.

In the drive for improvement in quality in the NHS, aimed at commissioners and providers, in 2013, Bevan proposed a three-way process for improvement including process, service and strategy innovations, using planned change which Bevan described as a road map. Within this paper, Bevan (2013) states the need for more than small changes, but that small changes can be used together to create larger change. By 2018, the NHS Improving Quality group (Bevan & Fairman, 2018), locating themselves in the emergent approach to change, were recognising a change away from hierarchical structures in the NHS and an increase in the speed with which change was occurring. The importance of networks is stressed to provide the influence required to make transformational change happen. They advocate that small change is insufficient to deliver 21st century health care, which seems to be at odds with the PDSA (plan, do, study, act) cycle of incremental change (discussed in the following).

Working across organisational boundaries is stressed to create a sense of shared purpose and shared values, included here Bevan and Fairman (2018, p. 8) note the need for 'emotional connections' to enable change. Within this approach, they advocate a change of emphasis from contracts and compliance to 'commitment to a common cause' (p. 8). They argue that listening to all parties involved will enable greater innovation (different ideas which challenge the norm) and greater commitment. Thus, the approach sets out ways of working rather than prescriptive structures, and acknowledges the emotional engagement needed to effect change. Readiness for change is acknowledged in the need for an organisation which ensures shared values and purpose, but one of the case studies used refers to being able to 'connect the disconnected' (p. 32). This suggests a judgement on those who are not signed up to the majority view, rather than an understanding that emotional reactions to change can be significant.

We now look briefly at approaches in North America. The Canadian Health Service Research Foundation (CHSRF) considered the range of evidence-informed theories and models of change management available globally and devised an approach to manage change within the Canadian health care system (Dickson, 2012). The result was a practical model for change management encompassing three stages: planning, implementing, and spreading and sustaining change. Antwi and Kale (2014) conducted a review of the global literature and its relevance to health care and made further recommendations for Canadian health care. The first element of their recommendations focuses on readiness for change. Considerable attention is advised to a detailed environmental, ecological and legal analysis, along the lines of Lewin's force field analysis. Specific attention to the 'readiness of individuals and groups' (p. 25) in supporting change is emphasised. Antwi and Kale (2014) note the different interests likely to be present between the professional health care practitioners and those making the decisions as managers or at policy level and the importance of shared understanding of the change. Their advice to use process mapping as a tool to identify different views and find alternative solutions aligns with the NHS PDSA cycle. Within this they advise discussions with staff and patients, and use of a range of tools, to elaborate the detail of the issues. Considerable acknowledgement of the need for cultural change is evident, specifically noted is the need to shift towards a patient-centred approach from a traditional hierarchical system. Advice on how to implement change, and the difficulties of sustaining change are discussed. Thus, while there is significant consideration of factors which must occur before implementation of any change, the time and energy to effect and sustain change is seen as a challenge.

As a lever to focus on a change to primary care, Beasley (2009, p. 64) states that 'Healthcare in the United States, compared to other nations, costs far more and results in poorer overall population health'. She introduces the Triple Aim Framework, designed to improve patients' health and experience while reducing cost of health care per head of population. The significance of moving to a culture where different parts of the health sector work more effectively together in order to support the primary care focus is highlighted through a number of recommendations, including ways of working and use of technology. The drive to promote primary care is seen as a way to improve population health and therefore reduce costs. One of the stated components of this framework is 'a focus on individuals and families' (p. 64). This component includes working to improve practice through feedback from individuals (aligned to the PDSA cycle of the NHS), and giving patients and their families opportunity to voice their views in planning their care and taking control in managing their care (thus challenging the hierarchical nature of traditional health care delivery). The change in design of services to ensure better access is balanced by a way of measuring progress in health initiatives and to assess spending. It is an ongoing cycle. The framework is one in which regular review informs progress with the three aims. In this way it shows components of emergent change.

Quality improvement tools and techniques

We now turn to discussing quality improvement in healthcare and in particular, we explore the use of Lean methodology and the PDSA model of improvement. Quality improvement is an international activity and it is a key aspiration for healthcare organisations but the intent is not always clear, whether it is for financial saving, increased productivity or a genuine effort to improve the quality of patient care and the health of respective nations across the globe. In the UK, healthcare policy changes tend to dictate quality improvements through targets and incentives, in the main financial targets. However, Ham et al. (2017) have indicated that the government's plan for change lacks information on actual implementation. While there are many examples of improvement in healthcare across the world, the benefits of quality improvement methodologies are not clear or consistent in regard to cost savings, costs spent on improvement activities, patient health outcomes and satisfaction, staff satisfaction and benefits of change in healthcare processes. We neither have consistent data of the rate of success nor information as to whether these improvements have been sustained and for how long. Yet these methodologies continue to be used.

Quality improvement uses a variety of recognised quality improvement tools and techniques and methodologies. These range from Lean, Six Sigma, PDSA, Total Quality Management, Business Process Reengineering, Clinical microsystems and Experience-based co-design. The NHS England and NHS Improvement website has a lengthy list of improvement tools categorised by 'stage of project', 'type of task', 'by approach', 'by patient pathway'. The full list is overwhelming for any practitioners seeking to bring about improvement.

Alderwick et al. (2017) point to the many opportunities for improvement in the NHS and initiatives that have already been undertaken, those that are ongoing or could potentially be put in place to improve the financial health of organisations. They point to Timmins (2017) who sets out in monetary terms the amount that could be saved. However, though Timmins identified sums of money that could be potentially saved, the actual savings are not stated. Much of the language is about potential savings. The question of whether quality improvements can lead to financial savings was reviewed by the Health Foundation (Ovretveit, 2009). While the suggestion is that there are ample ways of improving quality and making financial savings, this has yet to come to fruition in actual savings for organisations. While there could be potential saving, Alderwick et al. (2017) notes this is not the purpose of quality improvement.

Popular in the literature internationally is 'Lean' methodology which emanated from the Japanese car industry. At its heart are two key values (Jones et al., 2021, p. 29) 'to make customer value flow and respect for people', giving weight to 'patient's central position to all activities and aims to eliminate or reduce activities that do not add value'. The Lean approach attempts to reduce waste at every stage in healthcare, be these processes, procedures, activities, tasks or jobs undertaken. Thus, everyone in the organisation from professional, technical, administrative staff to managers and executives, should take on the job of identifying waste in their sphere of responsibilities and get rid of anything and everything that does not add value to patients.

A recent report on quality improvement shared the stories of the 'journey' of quality improvements. Examples of the work undertaken by Trusts across the country were relayed, including the challenges, learning and solutions. The report concluded that quality improvement 'is not a magic bullet' and it is not an 'easy journey' (CQC, 2018, p. 37). Many of these NHS organisations have been working with the Virginia Mason Institute, a key proponent of Lean and a commercial company. While there are many feel good stories and much learning to be had, we do not have concrete details on cost implications nor similar data on patient health outcomes and satisfaction, staff satisfaction or outcomes of various processes. There is some data from individual organisations, but this is limited to one or two outcomes and with little evidence of sustainability. Considering the Lean methodology is so widely used across the globe and being used and promoted here in the UK, the important questions are: does 'Lean' methodology improve patient satisfaction and health outcomes? Does it make cost savings and increase productivity? Does it lead to staff satisfaction and are healthcare processes any more effective?

In a comprehensive review of 243 articles on Lean in health care, D'Andreamatteo *et al*. (2015) concluded that the evidence of Lean's achievement are not yet clear or consistent, despite the widespread use of this approach, with the US being the leader in the field and 'Lean' being used mainly in secondary care. Gosling *et al*. (2021) note that quality improvement activities in primary care are much neglected. Further evidence of Lean's role in quality improvement, and the lack of clear benefits, were ascertained in a systematic review of the literature. Moraros *et al*. (2016) examined patient health outcomes and satisfaction, cost savings, workforce satisfaction and process outcomes on applying 'Lean' and found no improvements in these areas and pointed to the adverse impact on staff. A more recent systematic review of Lean in healthcare, a global perspective, cites the many actual and potential uses and benefits of 'Lean' but its actual success in bringing about improvement in healthcare was not evident (Antony *et al*., 2019). With the engagement of commercial companies, not-for-profit and commercial consultancies in quality improvement and little evidence, if any, on sustained improved patient satisfaction and health outcomes, cost saving, increased productivity, staff satisfaction and healthcare processes, the question needs to be asked: is this money well spent?

The PDSA model, originating with Deming in 1983 (Deming, 2018) has been suggested as a tool beneficial for improvement in the NHS and a guide for this is available (NHS Improvement, 2018). The guide describes the PDSA model as one for 'developing, testing and implementing changes leading to improvement' (p. 2). The guidance specifically states that the PDSA cycle should be used in a way which prevents sudden and impulsive change, instead, trying out a change in a small way will enable data to be gathered which will enable adjustment to the change before it is rolled out into the wider organisation. It proposes that making changes in this way, through time spent on testing and trial and adjustment before full implementation, will reduce the disruption to the staff and patients involved. Donnelly and Kirk (2019), of the Wales Deanery, emphasise repeating the PDSA cycle in order to sustain change. The method of using small-scale implementation of change, so that the change can be quickly modified based on experience in practice before being adopted across the country, has been praised as well developed and integrated in NHS Scotland (Dayan & Edwards, 2017).

PDSA has been lauded as a 'powerful approach' (Reed & Card, 2015, p. 151) to improve quality and shape culture in health care organisations. While there are clear benefits in using PDSA as it was intended, Reed and Card (2015) highlight 'the multiple challenges of executing PDSA well' (p. 147). They cite the culture of health care as a barrier to successful change implementation, a culture which emphasises 'do, do, do' (p. 151) instead of one which invests in time and other resources to support the detailed approach needed for successful PDSA use. Thus, the clear insight of the PDSA model, which questions the rationale for successive changes which may not solve problems, appears not to be exploited due to the culture of rapid change in the NHS.

This focus on getting things done quickly, and the rate of change which occurs in the 21st century NHS, was also noted by The Health Foundation (Allcock et al., 2015). Their report suggests seven success factors for change at any level of the health system, one of these being leadership which engages staff. The focus of this leadership is described as 'the ability to engage people with a clear vision for change' and 'facilitating collaboration and sparking enthusiasm' (p. 10). There are some notable aspirations in the report, for example distributed leadership and the importance of 'staff feeling valued' (p. 14). The drive to eradicate the hierarchical approach to change is to be applauded. However, instead of questioning such a stance, the need for successive rapid change in the NHS is rather taken for granted within the report. Equally the need to assess the cost of change and the need to sustain change are neglected. There is little acknowledgement of the need to consider readiness for change in this report.

Failing to consider readiness for change can result in management following one direction and practitioners working differently. NHS Quality Improvement Scotland commissioned a study to improve clinical practice in the form of a change to perineal suturing technique following childbirth across Scotland. Page et al. (2008) describe this change and the 'ideological and cultural clashes' (p. 250) that occurred between management and those operating as autonomous practitioners. The study describes the planned change approach of managers, run hierarchically and with a step-by-step approach with assumptions made by managers that the existing organisation was working collaboratively. This suggests that any need to assess readiness for change had been overlooked by managers, and the need to give power to practitioners to enable enactment of change rather than take a hierarchical approach was not considered. In contrast to this was the very different and emergent approach to change operating through the practitioners who were used to the complex set up of different professionals and different ways of working. Thus, the practitioners experienced positive ways of working and shared this with professional colleagues in ways applicable to their working contexts.

A host of authors and experts have suggested there is much learning from previous or current improvement activities that could and should be considered in quality improvements. One aspect of interest that is of relevance to our new thinking on change management is outlined by The Health Foundation (Jones et al., 2019, p. 11). This is the idea of 'assessing readiness' for change, by this they mean 'the extent to which the organisation is both psychologically prepared for change (shown by the maturity of its learning climate), and has the right infrastructure, governance arrangements and leadership in place'. In our thinking we believe that in assessing the emotional and cognitive readiness for change, not only can we gauge the individual's readiness for change but the readiness of the organisation in which they work.

Summary

In this chapter, we have considered a number of theories, approaches and improvement tools for change management. We have identified that many of these have significant potential for consideration of readiness for change, including not just cognitive but also emotional readiness. However, the sense of haste and rush within the health service in the UK appears to detract from full use of the theories when applied in practice. For example, we noted that Lewin's theory is often reduced to the three-stage process, without sufficient attention to the remaining elements of the theory. We noted that Kotter stressed the need for time to make successful and sustained change, but time is not always given as a resource to ensure change is embedded.

There are healthcare specific models and we have explored these, including those from North America. These tend to be mechanical in their approach and, in the case of the NHS model, complicated with many elements and activities. Lean methodology and the PDSA cycle are popular improvement tools in healthcare. However, most reviews of Lean suggest little benefit to patient health outcomes, staff and patient satisfaction or improvement in processes. The involvement of commercial companies in supporting Lean in health care improvement needs reviewing especially when healthcare costs are rising and there are urgent needs to be met in healthcare, for example the health and wellbeing of the workforce. Use of the PDSA cycle is often simplified, so that its true value is not realised. For many approaches to change management in health care, the original method or cycle of change is oversimplified when put into practice to such an extent as to reduce rigour and effectiveness. While we recognise how swiftly many changes must happen, without time allocated as a resource and acknowledgement of the need for cognitive and emotional readiness for change, there is a real danger that change will be superficial and at least some individuals or teams will not change or will not maintain the change.

While research has shown that only some 30% of change is successful, in the NHS there is a lack of data on successful change and change failure and thus the national improvement agency must begin to address the issue of inadequate data provision, that is change successes and failures with details of spending, and give a clear steer on managing change effectively, keeping in mind that staff are the NHS's greatest resource.

The main thrust in current change management is based on changing how people think, that is the cognitive elements. Without enabling mechanisms to support emotional reactions to change, there is likely to be a block, and changing how individuals think will not be realised. If this emotional element is not attended to, then the cognitive engagement supported by many of the models of change will not be realised. Both emotional and cognitive readiness for change could potentially lead to successful change.

References

Abd El-Shafy, I., Zapke, J., Sargeant, D., Prince, J., & Christopherson, N., 2019. 'Decreased pediatric trauma length of stay and improved disposition with implementation of Lewin's change model'. *Journal of Trauma Nursing*, 26(2): 84–88.

Alderwick, H., Jones, B., Charles, A., & Warburton, W., 2017. *Making the Case for Quality Improvement: Lessons for NHS Boards and Leaders*. London: The King's Fund. Available at: www.kingsfund.org.uk/publications/making-case-quality-improvement

Allcock, C., Dormon, F., Taunt, R., & Dixon, J., 2015. *Constructive Comfort: Accelerating Change in the NHS*. London: The Health Foundation. Available at: www.health.org.uk/publications/constructive-comfort-accelerating-change-in-the-nhs

Antony, J., Sunder, M., Sreedharan, R., Chakraborty, A., & Gunasekaran, A., 2019. 'A systematic review of lean in healthcare: A global prospective'. *International Journal of Quality & Reliability Management*, 36(8): 1370–1391.

Antwi, M., & Kale, M., 2014. *Change Management in Healthcare, Literature Review*. Kingston, Canada: Monieson Centre. Available at: https://smith.queensu.ca/centres/monieson/knowledge_articles/files/Change%20Management%20in%20Healthcare%20-%20Lit%20Review%20-%20AP%20FINAL.pdf

Baloh, J., Zhu, X., & Ward, M., 2017. 'Implementing team huddles in small rural hospitals. How does the Kotter model of change apply?'. *Nursing Management*, 26(5): 571–578.

Bamford, D.R., & Forrester, P.L., 2003. 'Managing planned and emergent change within an operations management environment'. *International Journal of Operations and Production Management*, 23(5): 546–564.

Beasley, C., 2009. 'The triple aim: Optimizing health, care and cost'. *Healthcare Executive*, 24(1): 64–66. Available at: www.ihi.org/engage/initiatives/TripleAim/Documents/BeasleyTripleAim_ACHEJan09.pdf

Beer, M., Eisenstat, R.A., & Spector, B., 1990. 'Why change programs don't produce change'. *Harvard Business Review*, 68(6): 146–155.

Bevan, H., 2013. 'Three steps to a new innovation strategy'. *HSJ*. Available at: www.hsj.co.uk/technology-and-innovation/helen-bevan-three-steps-to-a-new-innovation-strategy/5064849.article

Bevan, H., & Fairman, S., 2018. *The New Era of Thinking and Practice in Change and Transformation*. London: NHS Improving Quality. Available at: www.england.nhs.uk/improvement-hub/wp-content/uploads/sites/44/2018/09/Change-and-Transformation-White-Paper.pdf

Bradley, S., & Mott, S., 2014. 'Adopting a patient-centred approach: An investigation into the introduction of bedside handover to three rural hospitals'. *Journal of Clinical Nursing*, 23(13–14): 1927–1936.

Burden, M., 2016. 'Using a change model to reduce the risk of surgical site infection'. *British Journal of Nursing*, 25(27): 949–955.

Burnes, B., 2004. 'Kurt Lewin and the planned approach to change: A re-appraisal'. *Journal of Management Studies*, 41(6): 972–1002.

Burnes, B., 2014. *Managing Change* (6th ed.). Harlow: Pearson Education.

Burnes, B., 2017. *Managing Change* (7th ed.). Harlow: Pearson Education.

Burnes, B., & Cooke, B., 2012. 'Review article: The past, present and future of organization development: Taking the long view'. *Human Relations*, 65(11): 1395–1429.

Burnes, B., Hughes, M., & By, R.T., 2016. 'Re-imagining organizational change leadership'. *Leadership*, 14(2): 141–158.

Burnes, B., & Jackson, P., 2011. 'Success and failure in organizational change: An exploration of the role of values'. *Journal of Change Management*, 11(2): 133–162.

Care Quality Commission, 2018. *Quality Improvement in Hospital Trusts*. Newcastle upon Tyne: CQC.

Chaboyer, W., McMurray, A., Johnson, J., Hardy, L., Wallis, M., & Sylvia Chu, F., 2009. 'Bedside handover: Quality improvement strategy to transform care at the bedside'. *Journal of Nursing Care Quality*, 24(2): 136–142.

Cooke, B., 2017. 'Bernard burnes: Choices, contexts, and changes'. In: Szabla, D., Pasmore, W., Barnes, M., & Gipson, A. (eds.), *The Palgrave Handbook of Organizational Change Thinkers*. Cham: Palgrave Macmillan. https://doi.org/10.1007/978-3-319-49820-1_68-1

Cummings, S., Bridgman, T., & Brown, K.G., 2016. 'Unfreezing change as three steps: Rethinking Kurt Lewin's legacy for change management'. *Human Relations*, 69(1): 33–60.

D'Andreamatteo, A., Ianni, L., Lega, F., & Sargiacomo, M., 2015. 'Lean in healthcare: A comprehensive review'. *Health Policy*, 119(9): 1197–1209.

Dawson, P.M., 2003. 'Organizational change stories and management research: Facts or fiction'. *Journal of the Australian and New Zealand Academy of Management*, 9(3): 37–49. Available at: https://ro.uow.edu.au/cgi/viewcontent.cgi?article=1223&context=comm papers

Dayan, M., & Edwards, N., 2017. *Learning from Scotland's NHS*. London: Nuffield Trust. Available at: www.nuffieldtrust.org.uk/files/2017-07/learning-from-scotland-s-nhs-final.pdf

Deming, W.E., 2018. *Out of the Crisis*. Cambridge, MA: MIT Press.

Dickson, G.S., 2012. *Evidence-informed Change Management in Canadian Healthcare Organizations*. Ottawa, Canada: Canadian Health Services Research Foundation. Available at: www.infoway-inforoute.ca/en/component/edocman/resources/toolkits/change-management/methodologies-and-approaches/resources-and-tools/1123-evidence-informed-change-management-in-canadian-healthcare-organizations

Donnelly, P., & Kirk, P., 2019. *How to Use the PDSA Model for Effective Change Management*. Cardiff University, Wales Deanery. Available at: www.walesdeanery.org/sites/default/files/How%20to%20Use%20the%20PDSA%20Model%20for%20Effective%20Change%20Management.pdf#:~:text=One%20effective%20change%20management%20model%20is%20Edward%20Deming%E2%80%99s,is%20a%20model%20for%20learning%20and%20change%20management.

Gosling, J., Mays, N., Erens, B., Reid, D., & Exley, J., 2021. 'Quality improvement in general practice: What do GPs and practice managers think? Results from a nationally representative survey of UK GPs and practice managers'. *BMJ Open Quality*, e001309. Available at: https://bmjopenquality.bmj.com/content/bmjqir/10/2/e001309.full.pdf

Greenwood, R., & Hinings, C.R., 1996. 'Understanding radical organizational change: Bringing together the old and the new institutionalism'. *Academy of Management Review*, 21(4): 1022–1054.

Ham C., Alderwick H., Dunn P., & McKenna, H., 2017. *Delivering Sustainability and Transformation Plans: From Ambitious Proposals to Credible Plans*. London: The King's Fund. Available at: www.kingsfund.org.uk/publications/delivering-sustainability-and-transformation-plans

Harrison, R., Fischer, S., Walpola, R., Chauhan, A., Babalola, T., Mears, S., & Le-Dao, H., 2021. 'Where do models for change management, improvement and implementation meet? A systematic review of the applications of change management models in healthcare'. *Journal of Healthcare Leadership*, 13: 85–108.

Hinings, C.R., & Greenwood, R., 1989. *The Dynamics of Strategic Change*. Oxford: Wiley Blackwell.

Jacelon, C., Furman, E., Rea, A., Macdonald, B., & Donoghue, L., 2011. 'Creating a professional practice model for postacute care: Adapting the Chronic Care Model for long-term care'. *Journal of Gerontological Nursing*, 37(3): 53–60.

Jones, B., Horton, T., & Warburton, W., 2019. *The Improvement Journey: Why Organisation-Wide Improvement in Health Care Matters, and How to Get Started*. London: The Health Foundation.

Kanter, R.M., Stein, B., & Todd, J., 1992. *Challenge of Organizational Change: How Companies Experience It and Leaders Guide It*. New York: Free Press.

Kotter, J.P., 1996. *Leading Change*. Boston, MA: Harvard Business School.

Kotter, J.P., 2002. *The Heart of Change: Real Life Stories of How People Change their Organisations*. Boston, MA: Harvard Business School.

Kotter, J.P., 2014. *Accelerate XLR8*. Boston, MA: Harvard Business Review Press.

Lewin, K., 1951. *Field Theory in Social Science; Selected Theoretical Papers* (D. Cartwright, ed.). New York: Harper & Row.

Leybourne, S.A., 2016. 'Emotionally sustainable change: Two frameworks to assist with transition'. *International Journal of Strategic Change Management*, 7(1): 23–42.

Liebhart, M., & Garcia-Lorenzo, L., 2010. 'Between planned and emergent change: Decision maker's perceptions of managing change in organisations'. *International Journal of Knowledge, Culture and Change Management*, 10(5): 214–225.

Luecke, R., 2003. *Managing Change and Transition*. Boston, MA: Harvard Business Press.

Maclean, D.F.W., & Vannet, N., 2016. 'Improving trauma imaging in Wales through Kotter's theory of change'. *Clinical Radiology*, 71(5): 427–431.

Mehrolhassani, M.H., & Emami, M., 2013. 'Change theory for accounting system reform in health sector: A case study of Kerman University of Medical Sciences in Iran'. *International Journal of Health Policy and Management*, 1(4): 279–285.

Moraros, J., Lemstra, M., & Nwankwo, C., 2016. 'Lean interventions in healthcare: Do they actually work? A systematic literature review'. *International Journal for Quality in Health Care*, 28(2): 150–165.

NHS England, 2018a. *Leading Large Scale Change: A Practical Guide*. Executive Summary. Leeds: NHS England. Available at: www.england.nhs.uk/wp-content/uploads/2017/09/leading-large-scale-change-practical-guide-executive-summary.pdf

NHS England, 2018b. *Leading Large Scale Change: A Practical Guide*. Leeds: NHS England. Available at: www.england.nhs.uk/publication/leading-large-scale-change/

NHS England, 2018c. *The Change Management Guide*. Leeds: NHS England Sustainable Improvement and Horizons Group. Available at: www.england.nhs.uk/wp-content/uploads/2018/04/change-model-guide-v5.pdf

NHS Improvement, 2018. *Plan, Do, Study, Act (PDSA) Cycles and the Model for Improvement*. ACT Academy. Available at: https://improvement.nhs.uk/resources/pdsa-cycles/

NICE, 2007. *How to Change Practice*. London: NICE. Available at: www.nice.org.uk/Media/Default/About/what-we-do/Into-practice/Support-for-service-improvement-and-audit/How-to-change-practice-barriers-to-change.pdf

Ovretveit, J., 2009. *Does Improving Quality Save Money?* London: Health Foundation.

Page, M., Wallace, I., McFarlane, W., & Law, J., 2008. 'Emergent change and its implications for professional autonomy and managerial control: A case study from midwifery'. *Journal of Change Management*, 8(3–4): 249–263.

Pettigrew, A.M., 1985. *The Awakening Giant: Continuity and Change in ICI*. Oxford: Blackwell.

Pettigrew, A.M., Ferlie, E., & McKee, L., 1992. 'Shaping strategic change: The case of the NHS in the 1980s'. *Public Money & Management*, 12(3): 27–23.

Pettigrew, A.M., & Whipp, R., 1993. *Managing Change for Competitive Success*. Oxford: Blackwell.

Pettigrew, A.M., Woodman, R.W., & Cameron, K.S., 2001. 'Studying organizational change and development: Challenges for future research'. *Academy of Management Journal*, 44(4): 697–713.

Phelan, D., 2010. *Best Practice Change Management Guidelines*. London: Procurement Programme. Available at: www.nhsemployers.org/~/media/Employers/Documents/SiteCollection Documents/Best_Practice_Change_Management_guidelines.pdf

Radtke, K., 2013. 'Improving patient satisfaction with nursing communication using bedside shift report'. *Clinical Nurse Specialist*, 27(1): 19–25.

Reed, J.E., & Card, J.A., 2015. 'The problem with plan, do, study, act cycles'. *BMJ Quality and Safety*, 25(3): 147–152. Available at: https://qualitysafety.bmj.com/content/25/3/147

Rosenbaum, D., More, E., & Steane, P., 2018. 'Planned organisational change management: Forward to the past? An exploratory literature review'. *Journal of Organizational Change Management*, 31(2): 286–303. https://doi.org/10.1108/JOCM-06-2015-0089

Sackman, S., Eggenhofer-Rehart, P., & Friesl, M., 2009. 'Sustainable change: Long term effects towards developing a Learning organization'. *Journal of Applied Behavioural Science*, 45: 521–549.

Sarayreh, B.H., Khudair, H., & Barakat, E.A., 2013. 'Comparative study: The Kurt Lewin of change management'. *International Journal of Computer and Information Technology*, 2(4): 626–629.

Sminia, H., 2017. Andrew M. Pettigrew: A groundbreaking process scholar. In: Szabla, D.B., Pasmore, W.A., Barnes, M.A., & Gipson, A.N. (eds.), *The Palgrave Handbook of Organizational Change Thinkers*. London: Palgrave Macmillan.

Stetler, C.B., Ritchie, J., Rycroft-Malone, J, Schultz, A., & Charns, M., 2007. 'Improving quality of care through routine, successful implementation of evidence-based practice at the bedside: An organizational case study protocol using the Pettigrew and Whipp model of strategic change'. *Implementation Science*, 2(3): 1–13. Available at: https://implementationscience.biomedcentral.com/articles/10.1186/1748-5908-2-3

Suc, J., Prokosch, H.-U., & Ganslandt, T., 2009. 'Applicability of Lewin's change management model in a hospital setting'. *Methods of information in medicine*, 48(5): 419–428.

Sutherland, K., 2013. 'Applying Lewin's change management theory to the implementation of bar-coded medication administration'. *Canadian Journal of Nursing Informatics*, 8: 1–2.

Teixeira, B., & Austin, Z., 2017. 'How are pharmacists in Ontario adapting to practice change? Results of a qualitative analysis using Kotter's change management model'. *Canadian Pharmacy Journal*, 150(3): 198–205.

Timmins, N., 2017. *Tackling Variations in Clinical Care*. London: The King's Fund. Available at: www.kingsfund.org.uk/sites/default/files/field/field_publication_file/Getting_it_right_Kings_Fund_June_2017.pdf

Tinkler, M., Hoy, L., & Martin, D., 2014. 'A framework for challenging deficits in compression bandaging techniques'. *British Journal of Community Nursing*, 19(suppl. 9): S14–S21.

4
CRITIQUE OF CHANGE MANAGEMENT APPROACHES

Behavioural and emotionally centred models

Introduction

The gamut of approaches to change management have largely been developed with the emphasis on influencing people's thinking about change. The language and tone of these models and approaches is often technical, almost robotic in persuading people to accept and work with change. In this chapter, we explore a number of other models that are not frequently reported in managing organisational or practice change in health care. These approaches are important because they focus on emotion which Goleman (2006) describes as one of our two minds. The number of these approaches to change is not large, hence this chapter is shorter. We have argued in this book that we do not function with either emotion or cognition but with both. An awareness of the range of change approaches can be valuable for practitioners and change leaders to enable greater insight into how change affects people and how change can be implemented more effectively. There may be occasions when the focus for change will be on emotions, though to address emotions and not cognition is to neglect the entirety of human nature. Exploring these theories presents change leaders with the opportunity to critically evaluate the wide range of change approaches to help with their decision making on how best to manage change and see our rationale that effective change is potentially through emotional and cognitive readiness for change.

The models here largely emanate from the field of psychology and behavioural science. Positive reinforcement has long been identified as important to not only change behaviour but also to maintain such change, several approaches are included here and have been used to change both individual and organisational behaviours. We touch again on Lewin's model here, but this is discussed in more detail in Chapter 3. Kübler Ross's work on the grief cycle and Bridges' Transition Model are explored. Both of these see emotion at the heart of the change process

DOI: 10.4324/9781003128397-4

that people experience while Appreciative Inquiry focuses on the positive factors already present in organisations or groups to improve situations. We next explore behavioural and cognitive theories and consider a number of works including those of McGregor, Bandura, Maslow and Rogers. Finally, we wanted to consider theories specific to health behaviour and explore two theories within the health context that focus on changing the health behaviour of individuals and populations. Thus, we end this section with an exploration of the Nudge theory and the Transtheoretical Change Model.

The link between sensemaking and emotion is drawn out in this chapter, recognising that cognition and emotion are not separate from each other but interlinked.

Emotion at the heart of change

In Chapter 3, we saw that Lewin's model is considered a fundamental one in change management. Successive writers have diminished Lewin's original work suggesting it to be too simplistic for the modern world of constant change and complexity (e.g. reducing it to the simple three stages, without the element of group dynamics and force field analysis), while still referring to his work as the classic model of change. Cummings *et al.* (2016) critique of this was referred to in Chapter 3. The group is all important to Lewin (Lewin, 1951), he sees that the individual is unable to act alone due to the pressure of the group. The emphasis in his model is not the individuals which make up the group, each of whom may be experiencing different emotions, but the group itself as it exerts influence over its members. Burnes (2004) notes, however, that Lewin developed a process of Action Research to enable change in organisations which enabled the people to be involved in considering the situation, and considering options for change, and planning for such change. Action Research must be 'participative and collaborative' (Burnes, 2004, p. 984). In other words, the original ideas of Lewin, effecting change by working through group dynamics and force field analysis in a structure of Action Research through a three-stage process, took account of people as they functioned within groups. But over time, this emphasis on people has often been lost from what is now presented to practitioners as Lewin's model. For example, Kaminski (2011) provides a very clear summary of Lewin's three stages of unfreezing, changing and refreezing, and a diagram of different forces at work within a force field analysis, but does not identify the people and their important roles in change. Furthermore, the individual emotional responses to change, which will impact on group dynamics, are not considered.

Within the UK, the NHS is just one of the public sector organisations which has been subject to relentless efficiency savings in recent decades. Leybourne (2016) describes the stress resulting from this, both at the top of the organisation and within the teams and members of staff affected. The push to achieve political objectives, through use of changing metrics, is often perceived to be at ideological odds with the purpose of the health sector as perceived by the professional practitioners (see Chapter 2). Thus, considerable stress is not unexpected when changes occur and emotions can be high. Three models have been selected to provide examples of the recognition of emotions in models of change.

Kübler Ross and change as loss

Elizabeth Kübler Ross is famous for her writings on bereavement, based on her work with people who were terminally ill and their loved ones. From a psychological stance, Kübler Ross identified a cycle of emotions experienced by the bereaved, often referred to as the 'grief cycle' (Leybourne, 2016). She described a series of phases, not necessarily linear, experienced when an individual is faced with the death of a loved one (Kübler Ross, 2009). Aspects of this model are now recognised as valuable in understanding how some individuals experience change as significant emotional upheaval, a process of loss of what was known and familiar and safe, and a requirement to move to something unfamiliar, unknown, where it feels unsafe. This emotional response to change can be linked to a higher staff turnover (Cunningham, 2006); clearly a concern in the health service where skilled, experienced professionals are vital.

The phases of the grief cycle include denial (not facing up to the fact that change is happening, an inability to cognitively engage with the changing situation), anger (an emotional response which may be directed inappropriately due to the strength of the emotion), bargaining (trying to find a way to maintain the status quo), depression (a negative emotion with a lack of energy) and acceptance (the stage of acknowledging that the change has/is occurring and being able to engage at a cognitive level once more). Any change, even if it is likely to have a positive outcome for the employee, can be experienced in a negative way (Leybourne, 2016). Typically, managers will focus on the process of change with a desire for a timely outcome. If they spend time on identifying emotional responses to change in their staff, and time supporting these staff through their emotional responses to change, this can be seen to slow down the process and delay the change. However, addressing these emotional responses to support staff can have positive effects on ensuring change occurs and there is no regression back to old ways. Davis identifies Kübler-Ross's work as a useful 'tool to support staff struggling with the change process' and a way to 'understand . . . reactions to change' (Davis, 2012, p. 273).

The popularity of Kübler Ross's work in supporting the management of change is evident in the way elements of the grief cycle have been incorporated into other models, for example Beer *et al.* (1990) who note that peoples' ability to cope is affected by major changes in the workplace. Thus, it can be a very useful component when planning change, recognising that different people will react to change in different ways. Taking these potential reactions into account, those initiating change could prepare staff to be ready when change occurs, they could create open communication with staff to ensure messages from staff are heard and considered in both implementing and maintaining change. Kübler Ross's model identifies very clearly that emotion affects cognition during grief. By extension, emotion can block the cognitive functions of employees when undergoing significant change.

Bridges transition model

Bridges (1991) explained that change is a process of transition and that managers must understand and work with transitions if organisational change is to be successful. These transitions are based in the individual's psychology. Bridges emphasised people in change and the emotional process of gradually adapting to a new situation or way of working. Bridges Transition Model identifies three phases:

> Phase 1 – Starting the process is a letting go of the old ways, described by Bridges as an ending. This phase is a recognition that something is indeed coming to an end and therefore there may be a sense of loss, discomfort, anxiety, unwillingness to change. Anger or other emotions are to be expected as the familiar is removed. The manager's role here is in supporting individuals and teams to let go of old routines and ways of doing things.
> Phase 2 – Described as 'shifting into neutral', this is the phase of moving to a different way of doing things (shifting). Energy is needed to help manage and cope with the change. The manager will focus on ensuring that what is happening and why it is happening, the message and the vision of change, are communicated to all those involved.
> Phase 3 – The final stage is one of moving forward as the change becomes established. The manager places clear emphasis on the new ways of working and provides rewards for those supporting change. Bridges (1991) describes this as a 'new beginning'.

Leybourne (2016) considers that Bridges Transition Model supports individuals with the emotional elements of change, which he argues helps to ensure the change becomes normalised, accepted as the new way of doing things. However, criticism of Bridges includes the focus on the immediate change and making it effective. Individuals may be experiencing change in many different ways, and elements of the change may affect the larger organisation or its ways of working with other groups, departments or companies. The impact of the change may be much greater than the immediate issue. The complexity of working within organisations such as the NHS is not well incorporated into Bridges Model.

Despite the identification of emotion with these two models (Kübler Ross's Grief Cycle and Bridges Transition Model), Leybourne (2016) argues both are underutilised and Woodman (2014) notes the scant regard given to the emotional elements of change. The challenges faced by those managers implementing change are also considered by Leybourne (2016) who questions whether the needs of individual employees as they cope with change are recognised by the manager, perhaps due to time constraints or a focus on the cognitive instead of the emotional. Managers, Leybourne argues, are driven by process rather than by people, what he describes as 'managerial intent' (p. 34).

Appreciative inquiry

Bushe (2012) traces the history of Appreciative Inquiry from 1979 in Cleveland Ohio, US, where doctoral students were investigating leadership amongst medical doctors. Cooperrider and Srivastva (1987) highlighted the limitations of action research, with its focus on problems to be solved, and Cooperrider undertook an 'Appreciative Analysis' (Bushe, 2012, p. 9) and went on to propose that instead of focusing on problems which required change, the focus should be on 'mysteries to be appreciated' (p. 9). At this point, Appreciative Inquiry was a research method aimed at generating new ideas rather than concentrating on problems. Srivastva led the way for Barrett and Cooperrider (1990) to focus on appreciation instead of action research as a means to leading change. The research method became recognised as a process for change during the 1990s as work was done with non-governmental organisations globally.

As a mechanism for change Appreciative Inquiry focuses on the positive, the existing strengths and opportunities that are already present in an organisation or group, and the importance of group members working together to use these existing strengths for improving, for changing the situation to make it even better. The cultural diversity of the group members may be hidden when organisational change is implemented. Appreciative Inquiry works with the diversity of the group members in identifying the strengths as perceived by the group. Appreciative Inquiry, like Lewin's model, is based in social constructionism and the notion that relationships and communication are fundamental to successful change. If it is to operate successfully within a social constructionism paradigm, the appreciation of what works well should be generated from the people involved, even if they have different views of what is effective or excellent. Through discussion a way forward will emerge.

Since its inception, a number of different methods have developed within Appreciative Inquiry, from four principles, to the 4D model, and since the late 1990s, the 5D model. It is considered as a mainstream method for OD (Bushe, 2012). The steps are as follows:

- Definition – Here the focus of the 'inquiry' is clarified. Effort is given to solutions and better ways of working.
- Discovery – Here, discussion enables past or present successes to be the focus of effectiveness and excellence.
- Dream – Possibilities for new ways of doing things are envisioned based on excellent examples of working practices from the past. Challenges to the existing ways of working are considered. Having a positive picture of the aimed-for future is essential to drive matters forward.
- Design – Here the planning for the change occurs, working with the group members to ensure all are involved.
- Destiny – As the design is implemented, progress is celebrated, the dream is being realised.

Despite the focus on the importance of communication and group work, Appreciative Inquiry is criticised for over-emphasising the positive, not enabling negative experiences or problems to be shared. It therefore has the potential to exclude those individuals who have different experiences to the majority, and not take note of the emotional challenge some individuals experience when undergoing change. Thus, the real issues may not be dealt with.

Behavioural theories

A large number of other theories exist which could potentially be applied to the management of change. In this section, we focus on just a small number of these theories to set the scene.

Psychologists tend to focus on human nature, motivation and needs. There are many key theorists who have provided valuable insights into human nature. How human nature is viewed by change agents is critical to their approach to change. McGregor (1960) developed his X and Y theory based on assumptions of how people behave. His X theory shows that human nature can be viewed negatively. It suggests that people not only have a preference for leisure instead of work, but are work shy and will resist all efforts to change and thus will need to be directed and coerced. Theory Y on the other hand, views people as self-motivators with a huge potential, with capacity for independent thinking, keen to take work-related responsibility and with the ability to reach great heights. Similar to Theory Y, other psychologists view people as having the ability to self-regulate, able to create worlds based on hopes and needs. There is general agreement that when human needs are met, motivation increases and individuals can make major achievements (Bandura, 1977a; Lewin, 1951; Maslow, 1968; Thaler et al., 2010).

Behavioural theories became popular during the 20th century as ways to support learning. They are useful in relation to managing change especially in relation to ensuring that a change will persist, and not peter out. Their main emphasis is that learning occurs through conditioning. Positive reinforcement of behaviour will increase the likelihood of a behaviour being repeated, negative reinforcement and punishment will reduce the likelihood of the behaviour recurring. When a change is introduced, managers could use positive reinforcement to establish new ways of working.

In the early 20th century, behaviourism became popular as a way of measuring how stimuli in the external environment can lead to changes in behaviour. Classical conditioning described by Pavlov explained that reflex behaviours could be associated with external stimuli. Skinner took this further in his descriptions of operant conditioning, linking external stimuli to voluntary activity rather than simple reflexes. Watson, meanwhile, suggested that all human activity was based in cognition.

Cognitive theories then developed to take these ideas further, considering the roles of attention and memory in learning and the way in which the mind constructs experiences into learning. Bandura (1977a) went further still with his theory of social learning. He emphasised the importance of learning through seeing others in action, through observation of people who were physically present, or through observing people's actions on film or through other media. He developed his theory to include learning through careful instruction of how something should be done. Bandura supported the notion of positive reinforcement, but whereas the behaviourists had focused on external reinforcers, Bandura recognised that intrinsic factors may act as positive reinforcement. He also described the importance of other factors if learning new behaviour was to occur. These other factors were: attention (avoiding distraction while observing); retention (remembering what was observed); reproduction (carrying out the behaviour which has been observed); and motivation (wanting to carry out the behaviour). Bandura (1977b) added the concept of self-efficacy to his theory, the individual must believe in themselves and their ability to act in particular ways, and this links to the importance of valuing staff and their actual and potential contributions if they are to respond positively to change.

Nudge theory also describes the importance of positive reinforcement in influencing the behaviour of both individuals and groups, but adds a different dimension. It is useful to consider this when the aim is to change individual or group behaviour. Alongside positive reinforcement, nudge theory uses suggestions, often indirectly, to encourage people to make relatively minor changes which have little cost and do not require much to put into practice. Originating in the field of economics, Thaler and Sunstein (2008) coined the term 'Nudge' in their book about how individuals and groups often make decisions which are not in their best interest whether for health, wealth or their own happiness. Such nudges occur through changes to the environment, which make it more likely that one choice will be made rather than another. A health care example here is the requirement to either opt in or opt out of organ donation. Opting in will require an active decision and a specific task, making organ donation occur only where the individual has taken this action. Opting out requires the individual to make a specific undertaking to prevent organ donation, so that many individuals will become potential organ donors through inaction.

Arno and Thomas (2016) evaluated the use of nudges to improve dietary choices by undertaking a systematic review of existing studies from what they describe as 'wealthy' countries. They found that problems of excessive weight continued, despite the numerous and often expensive initiatives which have aimed to encourage healthy eating or increase physical exercise. From their review, Arno and Thomas concluded that there was a 15.3% average increase in more healthy choices of food through the use of nudges. The implication is that nudges will not only encourage a change in behaviour, but because the change is subtle and easy, it is likely to be sustained. Such nudging could be potentially helpful for those working in public health, to encourage healthier choices across a range of issues such as encouraging physical exercise, reducing cigarette smoking, supporting positive parenting, as well as making healthier dietary choices. Supporters of nudge theory note the simple, subtle, inexpensive ways in which behaviour can be influenced.

They argue that people make irrational choices, which are not in their best interest, and nudging can be used to support healthier choices across society. One of the main criticisms of nudge theory is that nudges are in effect manipulating the way people behave, influencing their choices, somewhat paternalistic, and some would say removing freedom of choice. The person who makes the change to the environment is making a decision about which practice is better or worse than another. Van der Heijden and Kosters (2015) note, however, that this is little different to most public health policies, which determine the preferred choices and endeavour to encourage people to change to these preferred ways of behaving. Extending this work to managing change in the workplace, it suggests that managers can put in place 'nudges' to support staff to make desired changes in practice.

Staged models of change are also popular in changing health behaviours, such as smoking, dietary choices, drug use, and uptake of screening programmes. Prochaska and DiClemente (1983) originally described the transtheoretical model, the most popular of the stage models (Armitage, 2010), to support people in stopping smoking. Such models identify the 'readiness' of an individual to change their behaviour and encourage specific activities to enable greater readiness and adoption of the change. If the individual is not considering change, or is resistant, then intervention is considered of little value. The greatest value of the activities is linked to those individuals who are identified as ready to change, having made at least some attempt to do this (Horwath, 1999). Success with the model is seen as the individual's behaviour being changed sufficiently to impact positively on health and for this to be maintained over a period of at least 6 months, at which point the change is more likely to be retained. The model has been criticised for being unscientific, particularly in relation to the categorisation of stages (West, 2006; Armitage, 2010) but has also been found to be helpful to support more individualised rehabilitation, linked to the individual's readiness to change (Ekberg *et al.*, 2016).

Social Learning theory and Nudge Theory are based in cognition. The first engages in intrinsic reinforcement of behaviours which are desirable within a change process, showing how to enable easier learning of the new behaviours. The second is about manipulating the environment to influence change, to make change easier so that there is no effort involved on the part of the individual. The third model, the transtheoretical model of behaviour change, draws on both the rational and the emotional. The main way in which these theoretical approaches can be useful is when planning for the maintenance and continuation of an implemented change. They are rarely referred to in any models of planned or emergent change.

Taking a humanistic approach to human behaviour, writers such as Maslow and Rogers took the view that humans wanted to exert their free will and own their own development. Maslow's work (1968) described a hierarchy of human needs, where fundamental needs to eat, sleep and keep warm must be met before higher needs could be realised. His work demonstrates insight which can be useful to change managers. Maslow puts the need for belonging immediately above fundamental physiological, psychological and physical needs and below the need for esteem, creativity and self-actualisation. When a change is proposed, any member of staff who considers their sense of 'belonging' to be threatened is likely to function less well in terms of their cognitive and creative abilities. In the same humanistic vein, Carl Rogers (1983) described that people typically have insights into their own challenges which enable them to find solutions. Neither of these approaches tend to feature in studies of change management, but both identify that people have a role to play in facilitating change and that people tend to want to achieve their own potential. These theorists have influenced educational approaches, and the importance of being student-centred, quite widely. However, they have not played their role in engaging with employees to promote successful change.

The link between cognition and emotion

Rationality has been the prevailing philosophy in organisations, viewed as 'rationally ordered, appropriately structured, and emotion-free life spaces, where the right decisions are made for the right reasons by the right people, in a reliable and predictable manner' (Kersten, 2001, p. 452). Thus, emotion is perceived as irrational and unscientific whereas being rational is viewed as positive, coherent and goal orientated. Burnes suggests that organisations are not inherently rational, despite managers trying to present their decisions as based in certainty and logic (Burnes, 2014, 2017). Nevertheless, the rationalist view still persists (Rafferty et al., 2013).

So, are there any theorists looking at the emotional elements of change and how these link to cognition, and can these be helpful in understanding readiness for change? Steigenberger (2015) provides a useful theoretical approach to support understanding of how people try to make sense of change efforts in their organisations. He highlights that as change occurs, this disturbs the equilibrium and makes employees consider their individual situation, thinking about both the present and the future. Initial responses to change are likely to be subjective ones, reasoned in relation to the individual's perceived situation and their immediate view of how the change will impact them. Discussion with colleagues and drawing from available information will build a picture for the individual employee. Steigenberger describes this as the process of sensemaking and suggests that such a process will generate either positive or negative views of the proposed change, which will influence the outcome of the change. Sensemaking has clear theoretical foundations, which can be usefully applied to change management. Steigenberger argues, however, that this cognitive sensemaking is only part of the process because people will also have emotional reactions to change and these emotional components will influence their experiences and their understanding of the change.

We know from Shin et al. (2012) that change will be perceived more positively if the emotions experienced are also positive, and Maitlis et al. (2013) clearly link emotions to sensemaking, describing both positive and negative effects. Steigenberger (2015) goes further, identifying that emotion not only affects sensemaking, but that sensemaking itself can influence emotions. The work of Liu and Perrewé (2005) specifically looked at the role of emotion in organisational change, stating that negative emotions can be 'intense' (p. 263) but that emotions experienced by the individual members of the workforce may change as the change progresses. They highlight how managers should be conscious of both the cognitive and the emotional elements of the change process and should consider in detail how and when change is communicated when planning change, to maximise positive emotional responses and prepare the workforce to be in a state of readiness. A number of authors identify Lazarus' transactional model (Lazarus, 1991) linking emotion and change (Huy, 1999; Liu & Perrewé, 2005). This model considers that individual employees will initially decide whether the change is likely to have any influence on their own situation, dismissing any concern if not. However, for those individuals whose initial judgement is that they are likely to be affected, they will react in relation to their perceptions of the change to their work, their ability to manage such change and the likely outcome for themselves once the change is implemented. Liu and Perrewé used this to develop a cognitive – emotional model of how people react to planned change. They argue that initial responses to planned change might be excitement or fear, related to the nature of the information received and the anticipation of change. With further information and thought, emotions might change, but will be related to the individual's understanding of the way the change will affect their own situation. Different coping behaviours may be adopted, leading to emotions of 'happiness, pride, sadness, guilt, shame, frustration or anger' (p. 266) as the change and its progress are evaluated. Liu and Perrewé (2005) argue that the way in which information is communicated and the content of such communication will affect the nature of the emotions experienced by employees. Those employees who experience the emotion of excitement are more likely to be proactive in coping with change and more likely to experience effective change.

Much of the earlier discussion linking emotional and cognitive elements of change is focused on the period of time once the change has been introduced. However, it can be useful to anticipate the cognitive and emotional reactions to change, and create emotional and cognitive readiness in the workplace, something we consider in Chapter 6. In Chapter 7, we further explore and discuss the link between cognition and emotion and present the AC-W Change Management Model, designed to address emotional and cognitive readiness for change, which is potentially the key to successful change management.

Summary

We have demonstrated that there are many models and theories which could be drawn from when planning and implementing change. We have argued that elements of Lewin's model are very much focused on the people involved in change, but that this is often ignored by those implementing the change. Other models explicitly recognise that emotion is an important element of human behaviour, although such models are not always associated with change management, for example responses to grief and Appreciative Inquiry. Other models specifically identify change as a transition, based in human psychology, with emotion as part of that psychology.

A few of the models we have discussed attempt to change individual or population health behaviour. Nudge theory and the transtheoretical model are in this mould and attempt to draw on human psychology, however, the importance of emotion is not explicit.

It can be useful to draw from fields of work not typically considered when dealing with change, especially with maintaining change, and some of the behavioural and humanistic approaches to learning have been discussed in this chapter. While these theories are valuable in understanding human nature and enabling strategies to be put in place to help individual change, they tend to focus on emotion alone rather than emotion and cognition together. For change to be effective, both emotion and cognition must be recognised as influencing each other.

References

Armitage, C.J., 2010. 'Is there utility in the transtheoretical model?'. *British Journal of Health Psychology*, 14(2): 195–210.

Arno, A., & Thomas, S., 2016. 'The efficacy of nudge theory strategies in influencing adult dietary behaviour: A systematic review and meta-analysis'. *BMC Public Health*, 16: 676. Available at: https://link.springer.com/article/10.1186/s12889-016-3272-x

Bandura, A., 1977a. *Social Learning Theory*. Englewood Cliffs, NJ: Prentice-Hall.

Bandura, A., 1977b. Self-efficacy: Toward a unifying theory of behavioural change. *Psychological Review*, 84(2): 191–215.

Barrett, F., & Cooperrider, D., 1990. 'Generative metaphor intervention: A new approach for working with systems divided by conflict and caught in defensive perception'. *The Journal of Applied Behavioral Science*, 26(2): 219–239.

Beer, M., Eisenstat, R.A., & Spector, B., 1990. 'Why change programs don't produce change'. *Harvard Business Review*, 68(6): 146–155.

Bridges, W., 1991. *Managing Transitions: Making the Most of Change*. Reading, MA: Addison-Wesley.

Burnes, B., 2004. 'Kurt Lewin and the planned approach to change: A re-appraisal'. *Journal of Management Studies*, 41(6): 972–1002.

Burnes, B., 2014. *Managing Change* (6th ed.). Harlow, Essex, UK: Pearson Education.

Burnes, B., 2017. *Managing Change* (7th ed.). Harlow, Essex, UK: Pearson Education.

Bushe, G., 2012. 'Foundations of appreciative inquiry: History, criticism and potential'. *AI Practitioner*, 14(1): 8–20.

Cooperrider, D., & Srivastva, S., 1987. 'Appreciative inquiry in organizational life'. In: Woodman, R.W., & Pasmore, W.A. (Eds.), *Research in Organizational Change and Development* (pp. 129–169). Stamford, CT: JAI Press.

Cummings, S., Bridgman, T., & Brown, K.G., 2016. 'Unfreezing change as three steps: Rethinking Kurt Lewin's legacy for change management'. *Human Relations*, 69(1): 33–60.

Cunningham, G.B., 2006. 'The relationships among commitment to change, coping with change, and turnover intentions'. *European Journal of Work and Organizational Psychology*, 15(1): 29–45.

Davis, G., 2012. 'A documentary analysis of the use of leadership and change theory in changing practice in early years settings'. *Early Years, an International Journal of Research and Development*, 32(3): 266–276.

Ekberg, K., Grenness, C., & Hickson, L., 2016. 'Application of the transtheoretical model of behaviour change for identifying older clients' readiness for hearing rehabilitation during history-taking in audiology appointments'. *International Journal of Audiology*, 55(supp. 3): S42–S51. Available at: https://doi.org/10.3109/14992027.2015.1136080

Goleman, D., 2006. *Emotional Intelligence: Why It Can Matter More than IQ*. London: Bloomsbury Publishing.

Horwath, C., 1999. 'Applying the transtheoretical model to eating behaviour change: Challenges and opportunities'. *Nutrition Research Reviews*, 12: 281–317.

Huy, Q.N., 1999. 'Emotional capability, emotional intelligence and radical change'. *Academy of Management Review*, 24(2): 325–345.

Kaminski, J., 2011. 'Theory applied to informatics: Lewin's Change Theory'. *Canadian Journal of Nursing Informatics*, 6(1): 1210.

Kersten, A., 2001. 'Organising for powerlessness: A critical perspective on psychodynamics and dysfunctionality'. *Journal of Organisational Change Management*, 14(5): 452–467.

Kübler Ross, E., 2009. *On Death and Dying*. Abingdon: Routledge.

Lazarus, R.S., 1991. *Emotion and Adaptation*. New York: Oxford University Press.

Lewin, K., 1951. *Field Theory in Social Science; Selected Theoretical Papers* (D. Cartwright, ed.). New York: Harper & Row.

Leybourne, S.A., 2016. 'Emotionally sustainable change: Two frameworks to assist with transition'. *International Journal of Strategic Change Management*, 7(1): 23–42.

Lui, Y., & Perrewé, P.L., 2005. 'Another look at the role of emotion in the organizational change: A process model'. *Human Resource Management Review*, 15(4): 263–280.

Maitlis, S., Vogus, T., & Lawrence, T., 2013. 'Sensemaking and emotion in organizations'. *Organizational Psychology Review*, 3(3): 222–247.

Maslow, A., 1968. *Towards a Psychology of Being*. New York: Van Nostrand Reinhold.

McGregor, D., 1960. *The Human Side of Enterprise*. New York: McGraw-Hill.

Prochaska, J.O., & DiClemente, C.C., 1983. 'Stages and processes of self-change of smoking: Toward an integrative model of change'. *Journal of Consulting & Clinical Psychology*, 51(3): 390–395.

Rafferty, A.E., Jimmieson, N.L., & Armenakis, A.A., 2013. 'Change readiness: A multilevel review'. *Journal of Management*, 39(1): 110–135.

Rogers, C., 1983. *Freedom to Learn for the '80s*. New York: Merrill.

Shin, J., Taylor, M., & Seo, M., 2012. 'Resources for change: The relationship of organizational inducements and psychological resilience to employees' attitudes and behaviours towards organizational change'. *Academy of Management Journal*, 55(3): 727–748.

Steigenberger, N., 2015. 'Emotion in sense making: A change management perspective'. *Journal of Organisational Change Management*, 28(3): 432–451.

Thaler, R., Sunstein, C., & Balz, J., 2010. 'Choice architecture'. In: Eldar, S.S. (ed.), *The Behavioral Foundations of Public Policy*. Available at SSRN: https://ssrn.com/abstract=2536504 or http://doi.org/10.2139/ssrn.2536504

Thaler, R.H., & Sunstein, C.R., 2008. *Nudge: Improving Decisions about Health, Wealth, and Happiness*. New Haven: Yale University Press.

Van der Heijden, J., & Kosters, M., 2015. 'From mechanism to virtue: Evaluating Nudge-theory'. *RegNet Working Paper*, No. 80, Regulatory Institutions Network, Australian National University. Available at: https://openresearch-repository.anu.edu.au/bitstream/1885/71637/8/01_Kosters_From_Mechanism_to_Virtue_2015.pdf

West, R., 2006. 'The transtheoretical model of behaviour change and the scientific method'. *Addiction*, 101: 768–778.

Woodman, R., 2014. 'The science of organizational change and the art of changing organizations'. *Journal of Applied Behavioural Science*, 50(4): 463–477.

5
EMOTIONAL LABOUR AND EMOTION AND CHANGE

Introduction

Focusing on cognitive elements only has not been successful in bringing about effective change. A rebalance is now required. Emotion and cognition are essential elements for change as they have a symbiotic relationship, working in harmony with each other. Our rationale for addressing emotion is due to it being much neglected in healthcare literature. Its importance during change cannot and must not be underestimated. This chapter begins by exploring the nature of emotion. From a historical perspective emotion was considered a problem, going against good judgement. However, emotion is now acknowledged by psychologists as a vital component of action. Emotional labour is examined. We argue that the nature of caring already takes an emotional toll on health care professionals. Change brings an additional emotional burden and this needs to be given serious consideration when any change is proposed. We consider the literature on the impact of change on emotions within organisations and healthcare. We identify that change impacts the individual physically, emotionally, psychologically and financially, and can lead to many health effects and even disability. This is not a state conducive to successful change, quite the opposite, such a state creates so called resistance to change (see Chapter 6). Understanding and acknowledging the emotions of the workforce who will have to enact change can support positive and sustained change. The way in which change agents acknowledge emotion can benefit or stifle change. Change agents who take a negative view of human nature may blame employee resistance for a failure of change to take place, rather than considering emotion as an aspect of effective change management.

The nature of emotion: history, science and psychology

The question 'what is emotion?' is very difficult to answer as there is no current consensus. Biologists, psychologists, sociologists, historians and even computer scientists are amongst those interested in emotions. For us, the emotions associated with change are important, how people respond to and deal with change in terms of feelings, actions, mood, motivation to support the change and their sense of belonging and self-worth, as well as any health effects of change.

Philosophers identify passions with primeval drives, for example anger or aggression, which must be controlled so that reason can win through. To control passion, prudence, fortitude, temperance and justice were required (the cardinal virtues) suggesting the application of wisdom, self-control, discernment and a sense of fairness. Western epistemology was shaped by the belief that emotion needed to be cut out of the process of knowledge production. It is not possible to explore emotions without considering the historic perspective and its influence which still prevails and has a bearing on the way in which change is tackled in organisations. Some 27 distinct categories of emotions have been identified (Cowen & Keltner, 2017). Ancient philosophers viewed emotion as something that controlled humans as opposed to humans being in control of their emotions, whereas Solomon (2003) refers to emotion as the 'passion' and contemplated it in association with reason. Philosophy books (e.g. Stanford, 2021) tell us that Aristotle described emotion as something that affects judgment and the Stoics viewed emotions as pointless, while Descartes, a philosopher of the mind, saw a separation between the mind and body. However, a change in the perception of emotions emerged with David Hume (1711–1776) who gave emotions much needed deference (Schmitter, 2021) as did Fredrick Nietzsche (1844–1900) who state that more reason was to be seen in emotion than in reason. Some other significant philosophers in this mould were Edmund Husler (1838–1960) and Martin Heiddegar (1927–1962). There is no consensus amongst philosophers and psychologists on the conception of emotion.

The James-Lang theory (1884) posits that emotion is physiologically based. Thus, when an individual is faced with an event that leads to a bodily reaction, the emotional response is linked to the interpretation of the physical effects. However, the Cannon-Bard (1924) theory suggests that physiological changes and emotions occur concurrently. Thus, physical and psychological experiences of emotion work in tandem and neither are dependent on the other. Singer-Schahter (1962) alternatively suggests that there is first and foremost a physiological response, then thinking and reasoning occurs. It is the labelling and interpretation that leads to the emotion. Lazarus (1991) posits that an initial stimulus is followed by thought, producing both a physiological and emotional reaction.

The question that continues to be disputed amongst philosophers is whether emotion can be considered to be rational or irrational. As with any controversial subject, sides are adopted. Descartes and Aristotle were early philosophers who associated cognition with emotion and Solomon (2003) believes that cognition has a principal role in emotion. Cognition precedes emotion (Frijda, 1988) and Lazarus (1991, p. 353) suggests 'emotions cannot occur without some kind of thought'. Cooper and Sawaf (1997, p. 37) suggest that 'each emotion is imbued with its own signal or intelligence', in essence humans are in control of their emotion and use it 'always for a reason, always to communicate something'. Daniel Goleman goes so far as to identify that we have both a thinking mind and a feeling mind, which work together to influence our behaviour. Addressing emotion is about self-control, the essence of will and character (Goleman, 2006).

Kotter and Cohen (2012) suggest that the flow of see-feel change is arguably more powerful than that of analysis-think change. In other words, attention to emotional reaction to change could have greater impact than attention to cognitive aspects of change. Researchers over the years have been studying these areas and new thinking is emerging to help practitioners. Neuro-scientific and behavioural thinking have gone as far as suggesting that without emotional input, reasoning breaks down in relation to decision making (Damasio, 2003, 1999, 1994; Glannon, 2007; Churchland, 2007; Quartz & Sejnowski, 2002; De Sousa, 1987, LeDoux & Brown, 2017). The interdependence of emotion and cognition is an important consideration when planning and enacting change.

Emotional labour

The concept of emotional labour describes a practice whereby employees whose work involves contact with the public have to manage their feelings in tandem with their organisation's protocol in order to create 'the proper state of mind in others . . . the sense of being cared for in a convivial and safe place' (Hochschild, 2003, p. 7). Thus, employees try to show emotions based on societal and cultural norms rather than what he or she actually feels (Huynh et al., 2008). Arising from the notion of emotional labour are the concepts of surface acting, where felt emotions are hidden, and deep acting, where one tries to experience the desired emotion. Therefore, there is a mismatch between what is felt and experienced, and what is shown when engaged in a job that involves dealing with the public.

Emotional labour is a component of any caring role (Smith, 2012). Health professionals such as nurses are required to provide their work with a smile (Grandey et al., 2005). Balancing emotions is necessary, to suppress negative emotions (e.g. anger or frustration) and to display behaviour and emotions that conform to organisational rules, for example kindness or good humour in the interpersonal relationship with the patient (Badolamenti et al., 2017). Nursing literature has shown a growing interest in this type of emotional work and its physical and psychological implications (Leka & Jain, 2010). Evidence suggests that there is an association of emotional labour with aspects of poor physical and mental wellbeing such as stress, emotional exhaustion, depersonalization and burnout (Abraham, 1998; Schaubroeck & Jones, 2000; Brotheridge & Grandey, 2002; Bono & Vey, 2005). This has also been shown with work satisfaction (Van Maanen & Kunda, 1989; Ashforth & Humphrey, 1993; Tolich, 1993), work performance (Baumeister et al., 1998; Totterdell & Holman, 2003; Goldberg & Grandey, 2007) and turnover intentions (Côté & Morgan, 2002; Chau, 2007; Chau et al., 2009). When nurses' emotional labour engages with patients at a personal level, it has been reported to be satisfying, and job satisfaction is also achieved when feedback of appreciation is given by patients. On the other hand, when nurses' emotional labour constitutes demanding work, it could lead to burnout (McQueen, 2004). People who habitually evoke the stress of surface acting are more prone to depression and anxiety, decreased job performance and burnout (David, 2016).

But it is not only nurses who experience emotional labour, it is a factor that runs across health care practice. In her discussion of the challenges of practising family medicine in Canada, Dhara (2019) reflects on the needs of patients versus the expectations of administrators. The 'discrete demands' (p. 426) loved by administrators can be measured using targets and benchmarks whereas the emotional labour of the work cannot. She remarks that despite the ever-increasing numbers (of patients, of procedures) and increased throughput, this does not meet the needs of individual patients at their times of stress and 'doesn't necessarily translate to better medical care' (p. 426). While the proforma may indicate the need to refer a patient to another health professional, the physician knows that the best way to meet the individual needs of someone who needs to talk to their doctor is to have that conversation. She describes the work of emotional labour, with examples of therapeutic conversations with patients, as 'real work', exhausting work, but without recognition from administrators. The challenge of emotional labour is exacerbated in the UK by the drive for efficiencies, for example the pressure to reduce the 'length of stay figure' in hospitals (Bunting, 2020, p. 100) which shortens the relationship between patient and health care practitioner. Considering the debate between detachment and empathy in the work of physicians, Kerasidou and Horn (2016) note the challenges, stress and upsetting situations that physicians have to deal with on a daily basis. The authors identify that emotional labour is required to enact empathy, which in turn requires the practitioner to have self-awareness of their own emotions. However, this can be in conflict with the detached, 'professional' stance that may be perceived as expected of physicians and other health care practitioners. In other words, the emotional labour of the work is not only not recognised, but not valued, so that training opportunities are missed. In their narrative review, Badolamenti et al. (2017) describe the importance to the wellbeing of health care staff of having the emotional labour of their work recognised and in their review paper, Riley and Weiss (2015) sought to better understand emotional labour in health care settings and through this to identify training needs. They found that emotional labour occurred not just in relation to the health care worker's role in caring for patients, but also in their interactions with the multidisciplinary team and in facing demands from the organisation. They also found that emotional labour was frequently undervalued by managers, and that staff will show resistance to change if they perceive that the emotional labour of their work is not valued, suggesting that if managers were to acknowledge the emotional labour undertaken by staff, resistance to change might be reduced.

A narrative review of literature from 2013 to 2018 to determine the impact of emotional labour on the health of workers in service industries, including the health sector, was undertaken by Aung and Tewogbola (2019). They report workers experiencing health-related conditions due to emotional labour which affected the quality of the work done and had the potential to develop into long-term conditions, including 'burnout and fatigue to dysmenorrhea, disruptions in sleep patterns and suicidal tendencies' (p. 273). They note the impact this could have on productivity and recommend that managers acknowledge the emotional labour of the work of employees and support them in this aspect of their work. One way of doing this could be by supporting the development of emotional intelligence in their workforce (Psilopanagioti et al., 2012). These authors considered the surface acting element of physicians' emotional labour alongside emotional intelligence. For the surface acting component of emotional labour, the correlation with job satisfaction was negative. They found that the surface acting component was linked to stress and anxiety and depression. On the other hand, they drew the conclusion that those physicians with higher emotional intelligence had better job satisfaction, emotional intelligence acted as an asset when having to undertake surface acting, suggesting that attention to development of emotional intelligence could have beneficial effects with respect to emotional labour.

We have seen that emotional labour is an important aspect of health care roles. While this can be both a rewarding and satisfying part of the work, it can be demanding and lead to physical and mental ill effects for the health care professional. Acknowledgement of this element of caring by health care managers is limited and can cause conflict within the workplace. With the added burden of emotional labour, health care professionals need a voice on how best to manage change.

Emotional impact of change

Change has been a feature of health care, the business world and in particular the NHS, which has been undergoing continuous change since its creation. Yet the literature on the impact of change in the NHS and healthcare in general is surprisingly limited considering healthcare is a large industry globally and the NHS in particular is the largest employer in Europe. We consider the literature on the impact of change in organisations and within healthcare here and in various sections of this book in Chapters 4, 6, 7 and 8.

Emotions are closely entwined with change (Jordan, 2004) and can determine the success or failure of organisational change (Daus et al., 2012). Change has a mainly negative emotional effect on staff and the emotions that arise can be intense (Piderit, 2000; Liu & Perrewé, 2005; Kiefer, 2005) reducing productivity and impacting negatively on performance. Feelings of being threatened, anger, fear, anxiety, cynicism, resentment, increased workload, job insecurity, withdrawal and poor organisational commitment (French, 2001; Conroy & O'Leary-Kelly, 2014; Begley & Czajka, 1993; Terry & Jimmieson, 2003) have all surfaced during change. Such strong emotions may affect those with a normally rational approach, so that relevant information is not understood as intended (Kirsch et al., 2010).

The grieving process may be experienced by those undergoing change (Holm & Severinsson, 2010; Giaever & Smollan, 2015). The uncertainty that change brings affects the morale of employees, their health, productivity and quality of care and leads to elevation of stress levels (Arnetz & Blomkvist, 2007) resulting in poor health outcomes, potential work disability and unplanned financial costs (Virtanen et al., 2010). Durdy and Bradshaw (2014) undertook a literature review on the impact of organisational change in the NHS with reference to mental health and concluded that change has a negative effect on staff. They note that positive experience of change is a rare event in the NHS because of the rate of change and poor management of change.

Health effects, including higher levels of occupational illnesses and injuries in workplaces during intentional transformations; increased stress levels; impaired sleep and recovery, have all been shown to occur in organisational change and to lead to poorer health (Greubel & Kecklund, 2011). Invasions of privacy, harassment, abuses of power and strong emotions such as aggression, resentment, denial, shock, anxiety, apprehension, cynicism and fear were experienced during downsizing, outsourcing, mergers, restructuring and continual changes, not only amongst individual employees but also managers (Smollan & Sayers, 2009; de Klerk, 2007). With regard to mental health problems, a review of the present literature concluded that there was not enough evidence to make a *causative* link between an increased risk of mental health problems and organisational change (Bamberger et al., 2011), however, poorer mental health, identified as increased levels of depression, anxiety and stress was found to occur in 11 of 17 studies which considered the impact of change on mental health. Further research is needed in this area.

Emotions do not always have a negative impact on change. Liu and Perrewé (2005) suggest the staging of emotions occurs with change, and that in the embryonic stage, a powerful range of emotions can emerge and thus may be the driving force for change.

While many studies consider the emotional impact of a single change, Klarner et al. (2011) researched emotional responses to multiple and follow-on changes in organisations. They are critical of the binary approach, where change is either seen positively or negatively, with negative stances being associated with resistance to change. This is too simplistic a view, change is more complex and employees may have mixed reactions and change is rarely a single event. In the modern world change is often relentless, with many changes occurring at the same time, and changes following rapidly on from each other. It is the culture of the organisation, and its ability to work with people during change, which must be considered. The views of employees in a range of industries were considered by Smollan and Sayers (2009), who focused on emotions experienced during change to the culture of an organisation. These changes to the culture included both intentional (planned) and unintentional (unplanned) culture change. The researchers demonstrated that where the culture matched the values of the employees, emotions tended to be more positive, but where the culture was at odds with that of the employees, emotions tended to be negative. Managers are encouraged to take the opportunity to develop an organisational culture which values the emotional labour undertaken by health care staff and accepts that emotion is inherent in change. The authors argue that attention to emotional responses of employees will draw positive reactions from them to enable them to work with the change. We consider readiness for change and engage with models of change that include emotional readiness in Chapters 4 and 6.

Staying with the theme of ongoing change, Kiefer (2005) describes that negative emotional experiences can be felt daily by employees, with staff worried about their future, their working conditions and the way they are being treated by their employers. With these negative emotions, the trust placed in the organisation is reduced and the individual becomes more withdrawn from the work setting. Giæver and Hellesø (2010) argue that too often negative emotions of change are linked to resistance, blamed on the individual and seen as irrational. These authors explored emotions experienced by nurses during the introduction of electronic care plans in a hospital ward. Their research did not identify any lack of willingness to change amongst the nurses, but there were considerable negative emotions related to the way in which the change was planned and enacted, with concerns about the lack of answers to questions about how to implement the system and the lack of training on how to use it. Giæver and Hellesø (2010, p. 44) state that 'The respondents felt very much left to themselves to work out how to solve practical problems in relation to the employment of the new system'. Thus, the negative emotions were related to trying to implement a change without the support of the managers who had introduced it and without adequate training. Their research also identified negative emotions related to the nature of the nurses' professional roles. The nurses in the study reported feeling that the new system was making their role more difficult and that they had to work harder to uphold standards of patient care. This suggests that the managers' role in change can be very important, with engagement of staff in the planning and implementation process, proper training, and a timescale for implementation of the change which is realistic.

On the theme of the impact of change at varying stages, Brown et al. (2006) examined the stress of nurses pre- and post-merger in the NHS and identified greater stress levels after the change. Smollan's (2015) qualitative study examined the personal cost of healthcare organisational change before, during and after change. He cites other prominent studies and voices across the globe on the impact of healthcare change concluding that change adds enormous stress on employees physically, behaviourally, cognitively and emotionally. In his own study participants reported effects in these same domains. Feelings ranged from anxiety, fatigue, anger and frustration to stress, which was exceedingly high in the transition period. Sleeping difficulties, headaches, individuals eating and drinking beyond the norm or not at all were noted. This fluctuation of emotions suggests that managers need to be mindful of not only changing emotions as change progresses but even when change is completed and ensure the provision of continued support.

Emotional intelligence and managing change

The previous section has identified that emotional intelligence can be useful in supporting change. But what is emotional intelligence, and how can it be used? In his 1995 book, Goleman explained that current definitions of intelligence were narrow, and that there were a number of attributes and abilities apart from IQ which contributed to success. Popularising the term 'emotional intelligence' he explained this range of other attributes. Included in emotional intelligence are notions of: self-awareness, the ability to recognise and control one's own feelings and emotions; resilience and persistence, having the drive or motivation and confidence to continue to pursue a plan even if challenges occur; being socially aware, able to recognise and react to different social situations and to use empathy to appreciate others perspectives; and finally to be able to relate to others through clear communication, appropriate influence and conflict management.

Many writers about leadership include emotional intelligence as an important aspect of an effective leader (e.g. Daft, 2011; Gill, 2011; Northouse, 2018) and comment about the way in which the cognitive and the affective domains are both recognised in notions of emotional intelligence. The emotional intelligence of leaders and managers has been linked to experiences of change management. Dhingra and Punia (2016) demonstrated managers who were self-aware and able to manage their own work and situation, in other words, who demonstrated emotional intelligence were more likely to demonstrate effective change management. In a Canadian study in health care settings subjected to numerous changes, employees were asked to rank their executive directors by perceived emotional intelligence and transformational leadership (Rinfret et al., 2018). The results showed that emotional intelligence was positively related to transformational leadership and employees linked this to a sense of justice within the work setting and a sense of job satisfaction. Such emotional intelligence is important across the health care spectrum, for example surgeons demonstrating emotional intelligence were able to enhance their skills of persuasion, manage situations of conflict better and manage change more effectively (Cavaness et al., 2020). Employees have been shown to be less cynical about change where the leaders demonstrate emotional intelligence (Ferres & Connell, 2004).

There have been arguments about emotional intelligence being largely related to innate personality traits, but a study by Vakola et al. (2004) shows that individual emotional intelligence separately contributed to receptivity to change. Their results show that those individuals who demonstrate emotional intelligence will understand the implications of proposed change and are more likely to react positively, whereas those without emotional intelligence will be more likely to react negatively to change. This is due to the way in which the emotions generated by change are managed by the individual employees. While there are other critics of the notion of emotional intelligence, it has become a useful concept to engage not just cognitively but also emotionally with leadership and change, and training in emotional intelligence is likely to benefit both employees and managers.

Training to support the emotional intelligence of teams undergoing change is recommended by Jordan (2005). Other studies show that health care staff use emotional intelligence in their everyday professional practice. For example, Kooker et al. (2007) demonstrated the use of empathy, and awareness of and nurturing of relationships by nurses. The nurses used their influence and acted as agents of change driven by their desire for good standards. These elements of their practice demonstrated autonomy and professionalism in their roles, which was often at odds with organisational practice, and led to nurses leaving the profession. With appropriate leadership, the professional practice could have been acknowledged and valued, rather than being seen as resistant.

Managing emotions in change

Research has demonstrated that part of effective management of change is to manage emotions, one's own and those of employees (Piderit, 2000; Steigenberger, 2015). Efforts given to management of emotions can contribute to managing change in a positive way (Steigenberger, 2015). A positive feeling heightens trust and thus commitment and emotional engagement while negative emotions can lead to mistrust and resistance (Klarner et al., 2011: Shin et al., 2012). Knowing that the wellbeing of people in their workplaces is connected to their emotional health (Department of Health, 2009), change management works best when all staff are given the opportunity to be involved, to work with planning and enacting the change which enables emotional engagement and trust to occur (West & Dawson, 2012; Ham, 2014). Positive emotions such as excitement enable staff to be optimistic about the change and cope with the differences which change brings (Shin et al., 2012; Avey et al., 2008). Fundamental to successful change management, therefore, is the quality of leadership in managing emotions (Fox & Amichai-Hamburger, 2001). Employing collective and distributive leadership will enable staff to be involved with the planning and execution of the change (Ham, 2011). Such leaders have high levels of emotional intelligence and are able to make best use of emotions in the work setting (Goleman et al., 2002; Antonakis et al., 2009). This emotional intelligence can enable the leader to see when the organisation is at a stage of readiness for change and can better help employees to adapt and work with the change (Norshidah, 2012; Huy, 1999). The effect on staff can be to worry less about job insecurity and be less stressed (Jordan et al., 2002; Ashkanasy & Daus, 2002). Critically, Goleman (1995, 2006) and others argue that training can improve emotional intelligence. Vakola et al. (2004) urge employers to take note, to set up training to enable emotional intelligence in managers and employees, so that change can be carried out more effectively. As part of such training to support change management in the organisation, they advocate developing skills in listening, negotiation, conflict management and motivation. They also advocate appointing staff who do not see emotion in a negative way but as a means to engage employees in identifying potential issues and working to solve such issues, thus supporting and sustaining change.

Having a network of support in work and outside could be in the preparedness plan of change for individuals to ease the stress of organisational healthcare change. Smollan's (2017) study on supporting staff during stressful organisational change indicates that 'support took various forms (emotional, instrumental, informational, and appraisal) and was sourced internally through supervisors and colleagues and externally through partners, family, and friends, at different stages of the change' (p. 282).

Summary

In this chapter we have considered different aspects of emotion and change. We began by thinking about definitions of emotion, and how ideas about emotion and its relation to cognition and action have changed over time. We concluded that current ideas about emotion stress the interconnection between feelings, understanding and action, so that attention should be paid to all of these if change is to be effective. We also considered emotional labour, and identified the considerable stresses placed on members of the caring professions in their normal everyday roles. Managers must acknowledge this emotional labour, and place value on it, if they wish these professionals to work constructively with change. Not only do health professionals expend emotional labour in their everyday work, but there is additional emotional impact when changes are imposed. We highlighted research which demonstrates that imposing change, rather than working with staff to generate effective change, can have poor outcomes.

Finally, we began to consider ways of managing emotions in change. We referred to the need for emotionally intelligent leaders who will work to harness what health professionals can bring to change rather than make negative judgements about resistance to change. Such individuals will lead teams who are ready for change when it occurs. There is a need for continued support from a variety of sources both within organisations and outside.

References

Abraham, R., 1998. 'Emotional dissonance in organizations: Antecedents, consequences and moderators'. *Genetic, Social and General Psychology Monographs*, 124: 229–246.

Antonakis, J., Ashkanasy, N.M., & Dasborough, M.T., 2009. 'Does leadership need emotional intelligence?'. *The Leadership Quarterly*, 20(2): 247–261.

Arnetz, B., & Blomkvist, V., 2007. 'Leadership, mental health, and organizational efficacy in health care organizations: Psychosocial predictors of healthy organizational development based on prospective data from four different organizations'. *Psychotherapy and Psychosomatics*, 76(4): 242–248.

Ashforth, B., & Humphrey, R., 1993. 'Emotional labor in service roles: The influence of identity'. *Academy of Management Review*, 18: 88–115.

Ashkanasy, N.M., & Daus, C.S., 2002. 'Emotion in the workplace: The new challenge for managers'. *Academy of Management Executive*, 16(1): 76–86.

Aung, N., & Tewogbola, P., 2019. 'The impact of emotional labor on the health in the workplace: A narrative review of literature from 2013–2018'. *AIMS Public Health*, 6(3): 268–275.

Avey, J., Wernsing, T., & Luthans, F., 2008. 'Can positive employees help positive organizational change? Impact of psychological capital and emotions on relevant attitudes and behaviors'. *The Journal of Applied Behavioural Science*, 44(1): 48–70.

Badolamenti, S., Sili, A., Caruso, R., & Fida, R., 2017. 'What do we know about emotional labour in nursing? A narrative review'. *British Journal of Nursing*, 26(1): 48–55.

Bamberger, S.G., Vinding, A.L., Larsen, A., Nielsen, P., Fonager, K., Nielsen, N., Ryom, P., & Omland, Ø., 2011. 'Impact of organisational change on mental health: A systematic review'. *Occupational and Environmental Medicine*, 69(8): 592–598. Available at: https://oem.bmj.com/content/oemed/69/8/592.full.pdf

Baumeister, R., Bratslavsky, E., Muraven, M., & Tice, D., 1998. 'Ego depletion: Is the active self a limited resource?'. *Journal of Personality and Social Psychology*, 74: 1252–1265.

Begley, T., & Czajka, J., 1993. 'Panel analysis of the moderating effects of commitment on job satisfaction, intent to quit, and health following organizational change'. *Journal of Applied Psychology*, 78(4): 552–556.

Bono, J., & Vey, M., 2005. 'Toward understanding emotional management at work: A quantitative review of emotional labor research'. In: Hartel, C.E., & Zerbe, W.J. (eds.), *Emotions in Organizational Behavior* (pp. 213–233). Mahwah: Lawrence Erlbaum Associates.

Brotheridge, C., & Grandey, A., 2002. 'Emotional labor and burnout: Comparing two perspectives of people work'. *Journal of Vocational Behavior*, 60: 17–39.

Brown, H., Zijlstra, F., & Lyons, E., 2006. 'The psychological effects of organizational restructuring on nurses'. *Journal of Advanced Nursing*, 53(3): 344–357.

Bunting, M., 2020. *Labours of Love*. London: Granta Publications.

Cavaness, K., Picchioni, A., & Fleshman, J.W., 2020. 'Linking emotional intelligence to successful health care leadership: The big five model of personality'. *Clinics in Colon Rectal Surgery*, 33: 195–203.

Chau, S., 2007. *Examining the Emotional Labor Process: A Moderated Model of Emotional Labor and Its Effects on Job Performance and Turnover*. Unpublished doctoral dissertation, The University of Akron, OH.

Chau, S., Dahling, J., Levy, P., & Diefendorff, J., 2009. 'A predictive study of emotional labor and turnover'. *Journal of Organizational Behaviour*, 30(8): 1151–1163.

Churchland, P., 2007. *Neurophilosophy at Work*. Cambridge, MA: Cambridge University Press.

Conroy, S.A., & O'Leary-Kelly, A.M., 2014. 'Letting go and moving on: Work-related identity loss and recovery'. *Academy of Management Review*, 39(1): 67–87.

Cooper, R., & Sawaf, A., 1997. *Emotional Intelligence in Leadership and Organisations*. London: Penguin.

Côté, S., & Morgan, L., 2002. 'A longitudinal analysis of the association between emotion regulation, job satisfaction, and intentions to quit'. *Journal of Organizational Behavior*, 23: 947–962.

Cowen, A., & Keltner, D., 2017. 'Self-report captures 27 distinct categories of emotion bridged by continuous gradients'. *Proceedings of the National Academy of Sciences of the United States of America*, 114(38): 1–10.

Daft, R.L., 2011. *Leadership*. Andover: Cengage Learning.

Damasio, A., 1994. *Descartes' Error: Emotion, Reason and the Human Brain*. New York: Avon.

Damasio, A., 1999. *The Feeling of What Happens*. New York: Harcourt.

Damasio, A., 2003. *Looking for Spinoza*. New York: Harcourt Inc.

Daus, C.S., Dasborough, M.T., Jordan, P.J., & Ashkanasy, N.M., 2012. 'Chapter 14: We are all mad in wonderland: An organizational culture framework for emotions and emotional intelligence research'. In: Ashkanasy, N.M., Härtel, C.E.J., & Zerbe, W.J. (eds.), *Experiencing and Managing Emotions in the Workplace: Research on Emotion in Organizations* (Vol. 8, pp. 375–399). Bingley: Emerald Group Publishing.

David, S., 2016. *Emotional Agility: Get Unstuck, Embrace Change, and Thrive in Work and Life*. London: Penguin Life.

de Klerk, M., 2007. 'Healing emotional trauma in organizations: An O.D. framework and case study'. *Organizational Development Journal*, 25(1): 35–41.

Department of Health, 2009. *The Boorman Review of NHS Health and Well-being*. London: HMSO.

De Sousa, R., 1987. *The Rationality of Emotion*. London: MIT Press.

Dhara, A., 2019. 'Invisible work. Valuing emotional labour in family medicine'. *Canadian Family Physician*, 65(6): 426–427.

Dhingra, R., & Punia, B.K., 2016. 'Relational analysis of emotional intelligence and change management: A suggestive model for enriching change management skills'. *Journal of Business Perspective*, 20(4): 312–322.

Durdy, H., & Bradshaw, T., 2014. 'The impact of organizational change in the NHS on staff and patients: A literature review with a focus on mental health'. *Mental Health Nursing*, 34(2): 16–20.

Ferres, N., & Connell, J., 2004. 'Emotional intelligence in leaders: An antidote for cynicism towards change?'. *Briefings in Entrepreneurial Finance*, 13(2): 61–71.

Fox, S., & Amichai-Hamburger, Y., 2001. 'The power of emotional appeals in promoting organizational change programs'. *Academy of Management Executive*, 15(4): 84–93.

French., R., 2001. 'Negative capability: Managing the confusing uncertainties of change'. *Journal of Organizational Change Management*, 14(5): 480–492.

Frijda, N., 1988. 'The laws of emotion'. *American Psychologist*, 43(5): 349–358.

Giæver, F., & Hellesø, R., 2010. 'Negative experiences of organizational change from an emotions perspective: A qualitative study of the Norwegian nursing sector'. *Nordic Psychology*, 62(1): 37–52.

Giaever, F., & Smollan, R., 2015. 'Evolving emotional experiences following organizational change: A longitudinal qualitative study'. *Qualitative Research in Organizations and Management*, 10(2): 105–123.

Gill, R., 2011. *Theory and Practice of Leadership* (2nd ed.). London: Sage.

Glannon, W., 2007. *Bioethics and the Brain*. Oxford: Oxford University Press.

Goldberg, L., & Grandey, A., 2007. 'Display rules versus display autonomy: Emotion regulation, emotional exhaustion, and task performance in a call center simulation'. *Journal of Occupational Health Psychology*, 12(3): 301–318.

Goleman, D., 1995. *Emotional Intelligence: Why It Can Matter More than IQ for Character, Health and Lifelong Achievement*. New York: Bantam Books.

Goleman, D., 2006. *Emotional Intelligence. Why It Can Matter More than IQ*. London: Bloomsbury Publishing.

Goleman, D., Boyatzis, R., & McKee, A., 2002. *Primal Leadership: Realizing the Power of Emotional Intelligence*. Boston, MA: Harvard Business School Press.

Grandey, A., Fisk, G., & Steiner, D., 2005. 'Must "service with a smile" be stressful? The moderate role of personal control for American and French employees'. *Journal of Applied Psychology*, 90: 893–904.

Greubel, J., & Kecklund, G., 2011. 'The impact of organisational change on work, stress, sleep, recovery and health'. *Industrial Health*, 49(3): 353–364.

Ham, C., 2011. *The Future of Leadership and Management in the NHS: Report from The Kings Fund Commission on Leadership and Management in the NHS*. London: The King's Fund.

Ham, C., 2014. *Improving NHS Care by Engaging Staff and Devolving Decision-making. Report of the Review of Staff Engagement and Empowerment in the NHS*. London: The King's Fund.

Hochschild, A.R., 2003. *The Managed Heart*. London: University of California Press Ltd.

Holm, A.L., & Severinsson, E., 2010. 'The role of mental health nursing leadership'. *Journal of Nursing Management*, 18(4): 463–471.

Huy, Q.N., 1999. 'Emotional capability, emotional intelligence and radical change'. *Academy of Management Review*, 24(2): 325–345.

Huynh, T., Alderson, M., & Thompson, M., 2008. 'Emotional labour underlying caring: An evolutionary concept analysis'. *Journal of Advanced Nursing*, 64(2): 195–208.

Jordan, P.J., 2005. 'Dealing with organisational change: Can emotional intelligence enhance organisational learning?'. *International Journal of Organisational Behaviour*, 8(1): 456–471.

Jordan, P.J., Ashkanasy, N.M., & Hartel, C.E.J., 2002. 'Emotional intelligence as a moderator of emotional and behavioural reactions to job insecurity'. *Academy of Management Review*, 27(3): 361–372.

Kerasidou, A., & Horn, R., 2016. 'Making space for empathy: Supporting doctors in the emotional labour of clinical care'. *BMC Medical Ethics*, 17(8). Available at: https://bmcmedethics.biomedcentral.com/articles/10.1186/s12910-016-0091-7

Kiefer, T., 2005. 'Feeling bad: Antecedents and consequences of negative emotions in ongoing change'. *Journal of Organizational Behaviour*, 26(8): 875–897.

Kirsch, C., Parry, W., & Peake, C., 2010. Chapter 5: The underlying structure of emotions during organisational change. In: Zerbe, W., Härtel, C., & Ashkanasy, N. (eds.), *Emotions and Organisational Dynamism* (Vol. 6, pp. 113–138). Bingley: Emerald Group Publishing.

Klarner, P., By, R.T., & Diefenbach, T., 2011. 'Employee emotions during organizational change: Towards a new research agenda'. *Scandinavian Journal of Management*, 27: 332–340.

Kooker, B.M., Shoultz, J., & Codier, E.E., 2007. 'Identifying emotional intelligence in professional nursing practice'. *Journal of Professional Nursing*, 23(1): 30–36.

Kotter, J.P., & Cohen, D.S., 2012. *The Heart of Change*. Boston, MA: Harvard Business School Press.

Lazarus, R.S., 1991. *Emotion and Adaptation*. New York: Oxford University Press.

LeDoux, J., & Brown, R., 2017. 'A higher-order theory of emotional consciousness'. *Proceedings of the National Academy of Sciences of the United States*, 114(10): E2016–E2025.

Leka, S., & Jain, A., 2010. *Health Impact of Psychosocial Hazards at Work: An Overview*. Geneva: World Health Organization.

Liu, Y, & Perrewé, P.L., 2005. 'Another look at the role of emotion in the organizational change: A process model'. *Human Resource Management Review*, 15(4): 263–280.

McQueen, A., 2004. 'Emotional intelligence in nursing work'. *Journal of Advanced Nursing*, 47(1): 101–108.

Norshidah, N., 2012. 'The influence of emotional intelligence, leadership behaviour and organizational commitment on organizational readiness for change in higher learning institution'. *Procedia – Social and Behavioral Sciences*, 29: 129–138.

Northouse, P.G., 2018. *Leadership* (8th ed.). London: Sage.

Piderit, S.K., 2000. 'Rethinking resistance and recognizing ambivalence: A multidimensional view of attitudes toward an organizational change'. *The Academy of Management Review*, 25(4): 783–794.

Psilopanagioti, A., Anagnostopoulos, F., Mourtou, E., & Niakas, D., 2012. 'Emotional intelligence, emotional labor, and job satisfaction among physicians in Greece'. *BMC Health Services Research*, 12: 463. https://doi.org/10.1186/1472-6963-12-463

Quartz, S., & Sejnowski, T., 2002. *The Neural Basis of Cognitive Development: About How We Become Who We Are*. New York: Harper-Collins.

Riley, R., & Weiss, M.C., 2015. 'A qualitative thematic review: Emotional labour in healthcare settings'. *Journal of Advanced Nursing*, 72(1): 6–17. https://doi.org/10.1111/jan.12738

Rinfret, N., Laplante, J., Lagacé, M.C., Deschamps, C., & Privé, C., 2018. 'Impacts of leadership styles in health and social services: A case from Quebec exploring relationships between emotional intelligence and transformational leadership'. *International Journal of Healthcare Management*, 13(supp 1): 329–339.

Schaubroeck, J., & Jones, J., 2000. 'Antecedents of workplace emotional labor dimensions and moderators of their effects on physical symptoms'. *Journal of Organizational Behaviour*, 21(2): 163–183.

Schmitter, A., 2021. *17th and 18th Century Theories of Emotions*. Stanford Encyclopedia of Philosophy. https://plato.stanford.edu/entries/emotions-17th18th/.

Shin, J., Taylor, M.S., & Seo, M.G., 2012. 'Resources for change: The relationship of organizational inducements and psychological resilience to employees' attitudes and behaviours towards organizational change'. *Academy of Management Journal*, 5(3): 727–748.

Smith, P., 2012. *The Emotional Labour of Nursing Revisited* (2nd ed.). Basingstoke: Palgrave Macmillan.

Smollan, R.K., 2015. 'the personal costs of organizational change: A qualitative study'. *Public Performance & Management Review*, 39(1): 223–247.

Smollan, R.K., 2017. 'Supporting staff through stressful organizational change'. *Human Resource Development International*, 20(4): 282–304.

Smollan, R.K., & Sayers, J.G., 2009. 'Organizational change and emotions: A qualitative study'. *Journal of Change Management*, 9(4): 435–457.

Solomon, R.C., 2003. *Not Passion's Slave: Emotions and Choice*. New York: Oxford University Press.

Stanford, 2021. *Stanford Encyclopedia of Philosophy*. Stanford. https://plato.stanford.edu/.

Steigenberger, N., 2015. 'Emotion in sense making: A change management perspective'. *Journal of Organisational Change Management*, 28(3): 432–451.

Terry, D.J., & Jimmieson, N.L., 2003. 'A stress and coping approach to organizational change: Evidence from three field studies'. *Australian Psychologist*, 38(2): 92–101.

Tolich, M., 1993. 'Alienating and liberating emotions at work. Supermarket clerks' performance of customer service'. *Journal of Contemporary Ethnography*, 22: 361–381.

Totterdell, P., & Holman, D., 2003. 'Emotion regulation in customer service roles: Testing a model of emotional labor'. *Journal of Occupational Health Psychology*, 8: 55–73.

Vakola, M., Tsaousis, I., & Nikolaou, I., 2004. 'The role of emotional intelligence and personality variables on attitudes toward organisational change'. *Journal of Managerial Psychology*, 19(2): 88–110.

Van Maanen, J., & Kunda, G., 1989. 'Real feelings: Emotional expression and organizational culture'. In: Staw, B.M., & Cummings, L.L. (eds.), *Research in Organizational Behavior* (Vol. 11, pp. 43–103). Greenwich, CT: JAI.

Virtanen, M., Kivimaki, M., Singh-Mantoux, A., Gimeno, D., Shipley, M.J., Vahtera, J., Akbaraly, T.N., Marmot, M.G., & Ferrie, J.E., 2010. 'Work disability following major organizational change: The Whitehall study'. *Journal of Epidemiology and Community Health*, 64(5): 461–464.

West, M., & Dawson, J.F., 2012. *Employee Engagement and NHS Performance*. London: The King's Fund.

6
EMOTIONAL AND COGNITIVE READINESS FOR CHANGE

Introduction

The NHS is a large and complex organisation and we have provided some background and detail to this in Chapters 1 and 2. We have also noted the frequency of change in large organisations in today's world and the NHS is no exception. Some of the major changes in the NHS have been referred to in Chapter 2. Our concern is not just the frequency with which change occurs, however, but that these changes are often unsuccessful or have more limited success than anticipated. The success or failure of change has been linked to change readiness and this idea forms the focus of this chapter.

In Chapter 3, we explored a range of theories of planned and emergent change and identified the 'missing link' in many, a lack of recognition of the importance of considering emotional and cognitive readiness for change. Many of the theories and models have the potential to consider both cognitive and emotional readiness, but in practice it is common to find that the rapid rate of work in the health service means readiness is ignored. Where readiness is included, this is often limited to cognitive readiness, emotional readiness is not considered. The rationalist view of organisations still persists, and the vast majority of assessment of readiness for change focuses on cognition.

This chapter explores readiness for change, both cognitive and emotional. We start by discussing the notion of readiness as opposed to resistance to change, we consider what readiness means and how it can occur to make change more effective. We argue that effective leaders can prepare their staff to be in a state of emotional and cognitive readiness even when the next change is not known, and that such leaders will recognise the need for emotional and cognitive readiness each time a major change is to be implemented. Such leaders will see the workforce as a resource to support change, where their ideas and challenges have

DOI: 10.4324/9781003128397-6

potential for improved ways of working rather than the ideas of the workforce being seen as resistance. We introduce the AC-W Change Management Model and the accompanying tool for assessing emotional and cognitive readiness for change in its original form. We also include the revised versions of the tool for real time and prospective change.

Resistance versus readiness

We refer to resistance to change several times in this book and there is a body of literature which discusses resistance to change and the need for the leader of change to be skilled in conflict resolution. NHS publications identify resistance management as part of the change process (e.g. NHS Improvement, 2011). The term resistance suggests an active fight against the change by the workforce and can be unhelpful as it does not get to grips with the various reasons why employees do not embrace change, some of which could be usefully engaged with by organisations to make change more successful. For example, the known and existing structure within a workplace can be comfortable and familiar, change will alter this and introduce unfamiliar and often unknown quantities. Members of the workforce may be in the best position to see potential drawbacks or nuances of such change. There may be emotional reactions to such disruption as staff feel unsettled, but there may also be very practical issues to be considered if successful change is to occur. Staff and other stakeholders will want to know how the change will affect them individually as well as the nature of the change for the organisation. Individuals may have a real or perceived fear of losing something important, for example their current skilled role in which they are experienced, or the team with which they work. Will they have to retrain and form new working relationships in a different team? Change failure in health care practice may be connected to inadequate sensitivity to individuals' emotional reactions (Curtis & White, 2002), scant help with psychological adjustments (Baulcomb, 2003) and a lack of support and empowerment to adjust emotionally to service redesigns (Holbeche, 2006). Emotion is central to much of health care practice (Bulmer Smith, 2009) and change impacts psychologically (Verhaeghe et al., 2006). Klarner et al. (2011) note that strong emotions can lead to mistrust and to so-called resistance to change. Perceived individual resistance may be through fear, and fear can make it difficult for people to take on board all that is being communicated, so that individuals may have misunderstandings about the change. Here we see the link between cognition and emotion and the need to consider both in readiness for change.

Eriksson (2004) and Gill (2011) flagged up another reason why people may appear to resist change, the way in which change has been introduced and handled in the past and the success or failure of that change. Gill (2011, p. 21) cites a large study in the Philippines which demonstrated that when change management was poor, trust in managers declined and cynicism about future change increased. Rapid policy change, which is then reversed, can make a mockery of the way policy is made, for example the sudden creation of 28 SHAs in England and four

Directorates, with the Directorates then disappearing within 18 months of creation (Edwards & Buckingham, 2020). This does not engender trust in those in power.

Resistance to change may also relate to the abuse of positional power by those effecting the change. Daft (2011) notes that if power is not used appropriately, it will not be seen as legitimate, and employees will react by refusing to carry out instructions about the change or refusing to change ways of working. The notion of resistance to change is further challenged (e.g. by Knowles & Linn, 2004) because resistance is not the typical reaction of employees, it will only occur if the change is imposed in a way that appears to the employees to be unjustified. There are implications for leaders of change here. It is necessary for a leader to develop or redevelop trust before any new change will be seen positively by the workforce. It is also suggested (e.g. Ford *et al.*, 2008) that if leaders expect resistance then they will actively look for resistance and may interpret non-resistant behaviours in this negative way. Thus, a change of mindset in the leader is necessary.

As early as 1993, Armenakis *et al.* began to differentiate between readiness for change and resistance to change, with a focus on the beliefs and attitudes of employees, and their intentions, contributing to readiness. So called 'resistance' could in fact be useful information about how a change could be implemented more successfully if done differently with the insights of those doing the job. Choi and Ruona (2011) reconsider Kurt Lewin's view of resistance within a force field analysis. In this model, resistance acts as a restraining force, with employees seeing that the existing ways of working are effective and do not need to change. This can be viewed as cognitive engagement with a proposed change, and the employees may have very reasonable arguments which, if considered, could be used to adjust plans and make the proposed change more effective. However, these authors note that resistance is often perceived negatively by managers as being at an individual emotional level within their employees, where a person is blamed for not engaging with the change and labelled as resistant. Thus, genuine ideas about how to improve working practices to achieve desired organisational goals will be ignored.

A study in the US considered how hospital nurses experienced a change which had been imposed on them (Bartunek *et al.*, 2006). The study was unusual in that it considered the change from the point of view of those who were subject to it. The researchers identified that the nurses were not passive in receiving the changes but played different roles in 'making sense of them, having feelings about them, and judging them' (p. 203). Thus, there was both a cognitive and an emotional element to their experience. Their reactions could have been labelled as resistance to change, but Bartunek *et al.* (2006) found that the situation was far more complex. Some staff experienced the change as anticipated, others did not. Lack of involvement in planning for the change, and lack of explanation and training before and during the change impacted negatively on the feelings staff had about the change. In other words, a lack of opportunity for cognitive engagement impacted emotional engagement with the change. This throws light on the importance of openness from leaders, being open with their intentions, being open to criticism of their plans and being open to new ideas about better ways of working. It also highlights the importance of communication and training if leaders are to support both cognitive and emotional readiness rather than so called resistance.

In essence, the notion of resistance to change is generally unhelpful because it removes the opportunity to engage the workforce in planning for successful change.

Concept of readiness

Readiness for change was originally summarised by Armenakis et al. in 1993 (p. 681) as 'beliefs, attitudes, and intentions regarding the extent to which changes are needed and the organisation's capacity to successfully undertake those changes' and subsequent discussions of readiness have tended to use this original definition. Rafferty et al. (2013) unpack this definition and note that the first component, 'beliefs', includes both the belief that the proposed change is a necessary one, and the belief that the people involved and the organisation itself can carry out the change. This suggests that employees who are 'ready' will understand the need for change and see how it might improve organisational practice, it also suggests that employees will have sufficient understanding, the right skill set, and sufficient support from employers to be able to enact change. Much of this is about cognitive readiness. The 'attitudes' element of the definition appears to be seen by Armenakis et al. (1993) as fundamentally a cognitive understanding of why the change is being proposed rather than any emotional response which may occur as a result of the proposed change. The notion of 'intentions' in the definition is similarly criticised by Rafferty et al. (2013) as involving motivation, the willingness to work hard and expend effort to achieve a change. Such effort is unlikely to be expended if the change is not seen to be achievable or useful in improving the organisation's situation. Thus, the nature of the change and its relevance to the organisation, as well as the likelihood of success, are factors influencing employees' engagement with change.

There is still, however, no general consensus on the concept of readiness. Holt et al. (2007b) suggest readiness for change is about a state or process and sits on a continuum whereby individuals could be completely ready or not at all ready. Emerging from the traditional focus on cognitive readiness for change is an understanding of the role of emotional readiness. While it is important to rely on reason to support people to understand change, reason alone is not enough. Gardner (2006) describes the need for resonance, the need to engage with people's emotions, to help them to *feel* that the change is right. The original definition provided by Armenakis et al. (1993) has been revised by Armenakis and co-authors in Holt et al. (2007a, p. 235) which defines readiness as 'the extent to which an individual or individuals are cognitively and emotionally inclined to accept, embrace, and adopt' change.

Theorising organisational readiness for change, Weiner (2009) notes that readiness will vary depending on the value which each member of the workforce gives to the change alongside a realistic assessment by the workforce of the potential for the change to succeed given the current situation, the resources and the expectations. He notes that it is not easy to bring this readiness across the organisation. However, if the organisation is ready for change, then the individual members of the workforce are more likely to put effort into making the change and making a success of the change, thus the change is more likely to succeed.

Undertaking a theoretical review of the literature on readiness for change, and describing change readiness as the 'most prevalent positive attitude toward change' (p. 111), Rafferty et al. (2013) found agreement amongst researchers on ideas about cognitive readiness for change, but a dearth of work about emotional readiness for change. Their review highlights how attitudes have both knowledge-based and emotionally based components, and that both components must be incorporated into any consideration of readiness as both will impact on behaviour. Rafferty et al. (2013) were also critical of the lack of 'multilevel perspective' (p. 110) when considering readiness for change. They found that much of the research about readiness was about individual readiness for change, and that this had been extrapolated to reflect group responses and organisational change without considering the different factors operating at the different levels.

Writing from a human resource perspective, Choi and Ruona (2011) highlight early ideas about readiness, linked to changes in individual health behaviours such as cessation of cigarette smoking. They argue that such changes in personal behaviour are based on the person's perceived need for the change alongside the individual's belief in their ability to change (as in the transtheoretical model described in Chapter 4). At an individual level, a person is in a state of readiness to change when 'he/she exhibits a proactive and positive attitude that can be translated into willingness to support and confidence in succeeding in such an initiative' (Vakola, 2013, p. 98). This does not mean a blind acceptance, as different factors about the change itself will influence attitudes, but it does imply an openness to ideas about change. At the group level, there is recognition that there can be peer influence, and sharing accurate information between members of the team rather than allowing for hearsay to spread is important. Change leaders take note! Applying readiness to the organisational level, the individuals concerned will seek out available information about the change, and make assumptions based on this information and their own situation and experience. The individuals will make a judgement about their own and the organisation's ability to change alongside a judgement about whether the change is perceived as necessary. Thus, individuals will have a sense of their own readiness to be part of an organisational change and also a sense of whether the organisation is ready for the change. This argument presents the individual employees as active in understanding their own and others readiness to change rather than as passive recipients of change or resistors of change. In this way, rather than seeing employee concerns about change as resistance, leaders can see them as genuine and useful concerns which need to be addressed.

The aforementioned argument indicates that the organisation can do much to be in a state of readiness for change. Choi and Ruona (2011) link readiness for change with Kurt Lewin's 'unfreezing' in the change process, a precursor to any change, and suggest this is a much more useful way to consider individual responses to change than the concept of resistance. By harnessing the ideas and concerns of the workforce within the organisation, such concerns can be considered and addressed, to provide a solution in which the change can be, and can be perceived to be, both positive and necessary. Such ways of working, to establish a state of readiness at the organisational level, often require a new culture within the organisation, which requires leadership, communication, an acceptance that learning can occur at all levels and the development of organisational structures and systems of working. A culture of participation in change is likely to positively affect change readiness as employees feel part of the decision-making process for changes which will impact on their work (Wanberg & Banas, 2000). Alongside this participation is the importance of communication throughout the change process, from planning phases through to implementation and embedding of the change. Effective communication can have positive effects on acceptance and outcomes of change, whereas lack of such communication can give rise to misinformation and cynicism (Rafferty et al., 2013).

We have seen that readiness for change has in the main been defined from a cognitive perspective, the ability to understand the change and the rationale for it, though emotional readiness is starting to gain ground. Rafferty and Minbashian (2019, p. 1642) report on two studies showing that change readiness is preceded by both 'cognitive beliefs and positive emotions about change'. Rafferty et al. (2013), in reviewing the literature on change readiness, suggest that more research is required around the role of affective responses and change. Emotional responses relevant to change readiness are many and various. For example, the emotion of hope may occur when a change is put forward, hope for improvements, hope for better working conditions, hope for better work-life balance, hope for promotion, as examples. Such hope is likely to have a positive effect on the individual's likelihood of embracing the change. On the other hand, an emotion such as anger may occur if a change is put forward which undermines the value of the employee or significantly changes their working conditions or work chances. This anger is likely to limit the willingness of the individual to embrace the change. Rafferty et al. (2013) argue that emotions in a work setting may be held at an individual level, but may also be held collectively, through shared communication in work groups or at higher levels of the organisation. Thus, the emotional climate of the work setting can be important in determining emotional readiness for change. This emotional climate is something which leaders can influence, creating a clear culture within the team or the organisation, developing team identity and developing trust. Unfortunately, some national guidance (e.g. NICE, 2007) can focus on the need to understand the change (the cognitive) and its desired effects, without regard to the need for emotional readiness for change. Other guidance identifies readiness as entirely focused on the manager or leader, with little or no reference to the employees and their contribution to readiness (NHS Improvement, 2011).

Steigenberger (2015) describes a theoretical approach, sensemaking, which links both emotional and cognitive elements of people's responses to change. We discuss this approach in Chapter 4. While it does not directly identify readiness for change, the theory is helpful in understanding that emotion and cognition are closely linked in responding to change.

Leaders' roles in creating readiness for change

Our discussion so far has identified that change readiness must be considered at the level of individual employees, work groups and the organisation itself. Writing about the 'unprecedented changes' facing the health sector and the need to consider readiness for change in terms of individual employees, Cunningham et al. (2002, p. 377) describe the way in which organisations are set up to support change. They identify that change brings emotional stress, and can lead to emotional exhaustion and undesirable health effects, and this can have a negative effect on patient care, especially where the job role is highly pressured. However, individual employees can see both potential benefits and potential risks of change and leaders should use this resource positively. These authors recommend leaders consider how the change might affect not only the individual's work role, but its impact on the outside life of the individual. They highlight the importance of individual employees' sense of self-efficacy and control over their own job, and the importance of organisations encouraging these employees to solve problem and be part of the plans for change. Successful change, therefore, is linked to self-efficacy, an individual employee's sense that they can work successfully with change but also that they have been part of the process to initiate or plan for the change. Such 'active involvement', reduces the stress of change and supports employees through the change. Leaders who promote self-efficacy in their workforce are promoting an environment in which emotional and cognitive readiness for change is inbuilt. Changing the culture of the organisation to both support employees to have this self-efficacy and to support a healthy working environment which includes the need for emotional wellbeing, it is argued, will enable the leader to support effective change. Where strong emotional reactions to change occur, managers are well placed to acknowledge that there may be good reason for such reactions, and to be able to listen, so that genuine concerns can be considered before change is implemented. Change can be stifled by managers who stick to a prescriptive model of change, which does not enable readiness (Stoller, 2018).

To enable cognitive and emotional readiness, and engage with the emotion of change, communication is fundamental. Leaders need effective communication throughout the change process (Durdy & Bradshaw, 2014), before, during and after the change, and an organisation which has effective working practices in place for communication is likely to be in a better state of readiness for change. For example, early accurate communication of proposals with the workforce will avoid rumour within workgroups, which can have a negative impact on understanding of and reception of any change. To establish such effective communication within an organisation is likely to require training, so that it becomes part of everyday normal work practice and will need to permeate throughout the workforce, and not be targeted just at one level. Change initiatives heighten emotions leading to people behaving irrationally and this in turn can impede communication through not hearing and understanding the change messages (Kirsch et al., 2012). Yongmei and Perrewé (2005) suggest that with the impact of change having a major effect on emotions, managers need to pay attention to the delivery and timing of change. Communication should be multi-faceted, so that there is an openness to enable the workforce to express concerns, put forward ideas and proposals, without fear of reprisal. Alongside this is an expectation that such expressions will be listened to and acted upon. In some cases, this will mean that leaders will need to adjust the change to make it workable. Such communication will also identify any specific training needs related to the change, and a timetable for such training will be required to enable the training to match the implementation of change. Training may also be needed in emotional intelligence (Jordan et al., 2002), which can help in understanding readiness for change (Norshidah, 2012) and can assist people to adapt to and facilitate change (Huy, 1999). This emotional intelligence enables leaders and members of the workforce to: manage their own and others emotions effectively; gain self-awareness; recognise the importance of persistence; understand the need for empathy with the local workplace culture; and develop strong and effective communication skills (Goleman, 2006). We discuss the importance of emotional intelligence in more detail in Chapter 5.

Preparation for effective change should include learning the importance of regular and repeated and detailed and effective communication with staff to improve psychological wellbeing and satisfaction at work (Terry & Jimmieson, 2003; Durdy & Bradshaw, 2014); considering the timing of change, and how and when the change will be communicated (Yongmei & Perrewé, 2005); considering how staff can be involved in decision making (Wittig, 2012); considering cultural change and the specific challenges which this will incur and how it will be enacted (Ham, 2014; Dawson, 2003; Cortvriend, 2004); and finally to consider how to ensure change will be sustainable (Martin et al., 2012).

A model for emotional and cognitive readiness

A potentially valuable model which encompasses both emotional and cognitive readiness for change is the AC-W Change Management Model. It can be conceptualised as a 'hub' and 'spokes' model. The 'hub' being the emotional centre of the model and the 'spokes' are the necessary conditions or anchors for effective change management in healthcare. This model has been designed with a trilateral purpose: assessing emotional and cognitive readiness for change; ensuring preparedness for change; and implementing the change. Change agents can begin change management by assessing emotional and cognitive readiness for change in their organisations, teams or departments. This will ensure the preparedness of people and resources for oncoming change. It is valuable to the organisation and the individual to undertake the assessment in different time frames. A tool to support the assessment of emotional and cognitive readiness is part of the AC-W Change Management Model and we include the original tool for retrospective assessment in Table 6.1. Therefore, the model offers the opportunity to assess retrospective change which will enable lessons to be learned from a change which has already occurred, so that a different approach can be identified for future changes. Prospective assessment relates to preparations which may be needed for a proposed change. We include the tool for assessment of emotional and cognitive readiness for prospective change in Table 6.3. Finally, assessment can take place as the change is occurring, in real time, to support understanding of how the change is working. The tool for assessment of emotional and cognitive readiness of a real time change is provided in Table 6.2. The tool has thus been adapted to assess for prospective, real time and personal change.

Throughout this book we have discussed the symbiotic relationship between emotion and cognition. In Chapter 5, we explored emotional intelligence. The work in this field has aided our understanding of how people function. We now know that both emotion and cognition are needed, and these two aspects interact to help with decision making. In Chapter 4, we discussed sensemaking, a theory that is helpful in understanding that emotion and cognition are closely linked in responding to change and in Chapter 7, we discuss further the interdependent link between emotion and cognition. More discussion on the AC-W model, with emotion at the heart of the model, and its nine spokes from which the tool was developed, is included in Chapter 7 with the use of the model and tool in case studies in Chapters 8 and 9.

Tool to assess emotional and cognitive readiness for change

The tool is a questionnaire, with open and closed questions, which can be used at the level of the organisation, the department or a smaller team. It is a simple-to-use resource for busy practitioners. Anonymity can be observed if required but in open and transparent organisations, anonymity should not be necessary. Ideally, the tool should be undertaken verbally with an appointed individual leading the change. There are advantages to this approach. It is an opportunity for face-to-face communication between change agents and staff and for change agents to encourage people to buy into the change. It is also an opportunity for staff to feel involved, engaged and empowered in the decisions on change management. Through engaging in this process, individuals are able to express their emotions about the change and this in itself can have a therapeutic benefit. It can further trigger the individual or the manager into seeking support for addressing any negative impact the change is causing. This human contact and dialogue between change agents and staff can lead to an emotional connection between staff, their work and the organisation which tends to benefit change management. There is a major drawback in this form of communication. Staff might feel constrained in setting out their views and opinions, for fear of being isolated, or being seen as resistant to change. Work might have to be done first to ensure there is trust in those leading change.

A potential criticism of using this tool is that it could be time consuming. Most of the questions used are closed questions, so relatively quick to answer, and this reduces the time taken for completion. However, we consider that time spent on assessment of emotional and cognitive readiness is central to change management. With change failure rates high in many organisations, it would suggest current change approaches are often ineffective in managing change and new ways are needed. Change relies on the involvement of the people in the organisation and use of this tool enables those people to be part of the change.

Use of the tool to assess emotional and cognitive readiness for change enables initial feelings, thoughts and opinions about the organisation and its opportunities and areas of development. Collation and analysis of the information provided will show the state of preparedness for change, from which a plan can be drawn up. Analysis may identify specific areas for training and development or may demonstrate the need for specific resources or expertise. For example, leadership development might be required, or putting in place guiding teams to support change. The extent to which staff feel involved in planning change, the effectiveness of communication systems, and the extent to which staff feel valued, either personally or as part of a team, will enable developmental work or structures to be put into place to support preparedness for change. The analysis will also show the extent to which staff consider previous changes to have been successful, where changes have been made and maintained rather than made and then lost again. Addressing these issues, planning to address concerns identified using clear goals, actions and a time frame, including required resources and training, will put the organisation in a better state of preparedness and support more effective change. Implementation of change can then take place.

The tools are presented here for you to use. Firstly, the tool for use when the change has already happened and it could be useful to discover how ready the organisation and its people were for the change (Table 6.1).

Secondly, we present the tool for assessment of readiness while a change is occurring in an organisation (Table 6.2).

Finally, we have included the tool for change which has not yet taken place (Table 6.3).

It is anticipated that by using these tools, a focus on emotional and cognitive readiness for change will enable far greater understanding of the issues involved in the change, and hence solutions which involve the workforce. This will lead to more sustained change.

TABLE 6.1 Tool for the retrospective assessment of emotional and cognitive readiness for change

Develop leadership skills across the organisation
Was there leadership in the organisation during the recent change?
Was this leadership evident across all parts of the organisation?
Was there a leader in your department?
Can you identify that person/role/position?
How did these leaders display their qualities and skills?
Did the leaders consider your feelings about the change?
Any other comments

Develop leadership and management skills of Guiding Teams
Were there Guiding Teams in place during the change?
Did these teams manage or lead the change or both?
What skills did the leaders of the Guiding Team display?
Did these Guiding Teams consider people's feeling about the change?
Any other comments

Build the right vision with inter-organisational wide engagement and involvement
Were you aware of the vision for the change?
Were you aware of organisation strategy?
Were you invited to meeting about the proposed change?
Were you consulted about the change?
Were colleagues or other professionals present at these meetings?
Were the feelings of colleagues and others considered?
Any other comments

Create inter-organisational communication forums in the frontline
How was the change communicated to you?
Were there forums for you to attend?
Were you invited to hear about the change?
Were there organisational partners or other professionals at these meetings?
Did change agents consider the feelings of these people about the change at these forums?
Any other comments

Create an empowering environment
Did you feel empowered in your organisation/department?
What would help you to feel empowered?
What made you feel disempowered in the organisation?
How did you feel when you are empowered/disempowered?
Any other comments

Create a culture of readiness for continuous change
How did you feel change should be managed in your Trust?
How did the organisation prepare you for new changes?
What preparations did you think you needed to be ready for new changes?
Any other comments

(Continued)

TABLE 6.1 (Continued)

Affirm and embed the direction of change in the frontline
How did you learn about the proposed change and what details were you given?
What preparations did you receive for the team/ward/department to support the change?
What preparations did your team members receive in order to sustain the change?
Was there regular support for you in maintaining the new change?
What would have helped to sustain and maintain this change in the frontline?
Any other comments

Develop organisational values that reflects the importance of all parts of the organisation
Do you feel valued in this organisation?
What makes you feel valued?
Do you think all levels of staff feel equally valued?
Any other comments

Use a model of change management that best fits the organisation's business
How was the recent change managed?
Were you aware of models/approaches/theories of change?
Did the organisation use a recognised model of change management?
Was it effective?
Were there areas that you would have liked the change to focus on?
Any other comments

Consider human emotions during the change process
How did you feel about the change?
How were your feelings addressed during change?
How would you have liked your feelings to be dealt with?
What other feelings did you experience during the change?
What would you suggest the organisation needs to put in place to address people's feelings during change?
Any other comments

TABLE 6.2 Tool for the real time assessment of cognitive and emotional readiness for change

Develop leadership skills across the organisation
Is there leadership in the organisation in the current change?
Is there leadership across all parts of the organisation?
Is there a leader in your department?
Can you identify that person/role/position?
Are leaders displaying relevant qualities and skills?
Are the leaders considering your feelings about the change?
Any other comments

Develop leadership and management skills of Guiding Teams
Are there Guiding Teams in place in the present change?
Are these teams managing or leading the change or both?
Are the leaders of the Guiding Team displaying relevant skills?
Are these Guiding Teams considering people's feeling about the change?
Any other comments

Build the right vision with inter-organisational wide engagement and involvement
Are you aware of the vision for the change?
Are you aware of organisation strategy?
Are you being invited to meetings about the proposed change?
Are you being consulted about the change?
Are colleagues or other professionals present at these meetings?
Are the feelings of colleagues and others being considered?
Any other comments

Create inter-organisational communication forums in the frontline
How is the change communicated to you?
Are there forums for you to attend?
Are you being invited to hear about the change?
Are there organisational partners or other professionals at these meetings?
Are change agents considering the feelings of these people about the change at these forums?
Any other comments

Create an empowering environment
Are you feeling empowered in your organisation/department?
What will help you to feel empowered?
What is making you feel disempowered in the organisation?
How are you feeling being empowered/disempowered?
Any other comments

Create a culture of readiness for continuous change
How do you feel change should be managed in your Trust?
Is the organisation preparing you for new changes?
Are you being prepared regularly for the change happening presently?
Any other comments

Affirm and embed the direction of change in the frontline
Are you being informed about the proposed change and what details are you getting?
What preparations are you receiving as a team/ward/department to support the change?
What preparations are your team members receiving in order to sustain the change?
Is there regular support for you in maintaining the new change?
What would help to sustain and maintain this change in the frontline?
Any other comments

(Continued)

104 Emotional and cognitive readiness

TABLE 6.2 (Continued)

Develop organisational values that reflects the importance of all parts of the organisation
Are you feeling valued in this organisation?
What is making you feel valued?
Are all levels of staff feeling equally values?
Any other comments

Use a model of change management that best fits the organisation's business
How is the change being managed?
What specific models/approaches/theories of change are you using presently?
Is the organisation using a recognised model of change management?
Is it being effective?
Is their specific areas that you would like the change to focus on?
Any other comments

Consider human emotions during the change process
How are you feeling about the change?
How are your feelings being addressed in this change?
How would you like your feelings to be dealt with?
What other feelings are you experiencing during this change?
What would you suggest the organisation needs to put in place to address people's feelings in this change?
Any other comments

TABLE 6.3 Tool for the prospective assessment of emotional and cognitive readiness for change

Develop leadership skills across the organisation
Is there leadership in your organisation for managing change?
Is there leadership across all parts of the organisation?
Is there leadership in your department?
Can you identify a person/role/position to lead change?
What leadership qualities and skills would you like in your leader?
Would you like leaders to consider your feelings about proposed change?
Any other comments

Develop leadership and management skills of Guiding Teams
Do you have Guiding Teams in place to lead change?
Would you like these teams to either manage or lead change or both?
What skills would you like leaders of the Guiding Team to display?
Would you like Guiding Teams to consider peoples' feelings about change?
Any other comments

Build the right vision with inter-organisational wide engagement and involvement
Would you like to know about the organisation's vision for any change?
Would you like consultation on any proposed change?
Would you like other professionals to be consulted?
Would you like the feelings of colleagues and others to be considered?
Any other comments

Create inter-organisational communication forums in the frontline
How would you like any changes communicated to you?
Would you like communication forums in place?
Would you like organisational partners and other professionals at these forums?
Would you like change leaders to consider everyone's feelings about change?
Any other comments

Create an empowering environment
Do you feel empowered in your organisation/department?
What makes you feel disempowered in the organisation?
How do you feel when you are empowered/disempowered?
What would help you to feel empowered?
Any other comments

Create a culture of readiness for continuous change
Is there an organisational change readiness plan in place?
How do you feel change should be managed in your Trust?
What preparations do you think you need to be ready for new changes?
Any other comments

Affirm and embed the direction of change in the frontline
What preparations and support would you like to help embed change?
What preparations and support would you like to help sustain change?
Any other comments

Develop organisational values that reflects the importance of all parts of the organisation
Do you feel valued in this organisation?
What would help to make you feel valued?
What would help staff at all levels to feel equally valued?
Any other comments

Use a model of change management that best fits the organisation's business
Are you aware of models/approaches/theories of change?
Would you like the organisation to use a recognised approach to change management?
How would you like change to be managed in your organisation?
Any other comments

Consider human emotions during the change process
How do you feel when change is proposed?
How would you like your feelings to be addressed?
What does the organisation need to do to address everyone's feelings when change is suggested?
Any other comments

Summary

In this chapter, we have argued that an organisation in a state of emotional and cognitive readiness for change will have greater success when putting changes in place. Employees are a valuable resource, with knowledge and understanding and expertise about their area of work and how change will impact that work. Effective leaders will harness that expertise and use it to inform the nature of change and the way in which change is implemented. Being ready for change is not just about having an understanding of the change. It is far more complex. In large organisations changes will have diverse and sometimes considerable impact on the ways in which teams and departments work. Using the valuable insights of health professional staff can support greater engagement with the change as well as more effective and long-lasting change.

The danger is that change is often seen by managers as a project to manage. The change is decided before it is presented to the workforce and the manager tells the employees what the steps are and what the outcome will be. Rather than thinking about change in terms of preparing the organisation to be in a state of emotional and cognitive readiness for change, the change is introduced with minimal involvement of staff who feel they are being told what to do without their insights being valued. Applying the AC-W change model enables cognitive and emotional readiness for change and could provide the energy, motivation and engagement for successful change management.

References

Armenakis, A.A., Harris, S.G., & Mossholder, K.W., 1993. 'Creating readiness for organizational change'. *Human Relations*, 46(6): 681–703.

Bartunek, J.M., Rousseau, D.M., Rudolph, J.W., & DePalma, J.A., 2006. 'On the receiving end. Sensemaking, emotion and assessments of an organizational change initiated by others'. *The Journal of Applied Behavioural Science*, 42(2): 182–206.

Baulcomb, J.S., 2003. 'Management of change through force field analysis'. *Journal of Nursing Management*, 11(4): 275–280.

Bulmer Smith, K., Profetto-McGrath, J., & Cummings, G., 2009. 'Emotional intelligence and nursing: An integrative literature review'. *International Journal of Nursing Studies*, 46(12): 1624–1636.

Choi, M., & Ruona, W.E.A., 2011. 'Individual readiness for organizational change and its implications for human resource and organizational development'. *Human Resource Development Review*, 10(1): 46–73.

Cortvriend, P., 2004. 'Change management of mergers: The impact on NHS staff and their psychological contract'. *Health Service Management Research*, 17(3): 177–187.

Cunningham, C.E., Woodward, C.A., Shannon, H.S., Macintosh, J., Lendrum, B., Rosenbloom, D., & Brown, J., 2002. 'Readiness for organizational change: A longitudinal study of workplace, psychological and behavioural correlates'. *Journal of Occupational and Organizational Psychology*, 75, 377–392.

Curtis, E., & White, P., 2002. 'Resistance to change. Causes and solutions'. *Nursing Management*, 8(10): 15–20.

Daft, R.L., 2011. *Leadership*. Andover: Cengage Learning.

Dawson, P.M., 2003. 'Organizational change stories and management research: Facts or fiction'. *Journal of the Australian and New Zealand Academy of Management*, 9(3): 37–49. Available at: https://ro.uow.edu.au/cgi/viewcontent.cgi?article=1223&context=commpapers

Durdy, H., & Bradshaw, T., 2014. 'The impact of organizational change in the NHS on staff and patients: A literature review with a focus on mental health'. *Mental Health Nursing*, 34(2): 16–20.

Edwards, N., & Buckingham, H., 2020. *Strategic Health Authorities and Regions: Lessons from History*. Research Report. London: Nuffield Trust.

Eriksson, C.B., 2004. 'The effects of change programs on employees' emotions'. *Personnel Review*, 33(1): 110–126.

Ford, J.D., Ford, L.W., & D'Amelio, A., 2008. 'Resistance to change: The rest of the story'. *Academy of Management Review*, 33: 362–377.

Gardner, H., 2006. *Changing Minds*. Boston, MA: Harvard Business School Press.

Gill, R., 2011. *Theory and Practice of Leadership* (2nd ed.). London: Sage.

Goleman, D., 2006. *Emotional Intelligence: Why It Can Matter More than IQ*. London: Bloomsbury Publishing.

Ham, C., 2014. *Improving NHS Care by Engaging Staff and Devolving Decision-making. Report of the Review of Staff Engagement and Empowerment in the NHS*. London: The King's Fund.

Holbeche, L., 2006. *Understanding Change: Theory, Implementation and Success*. London: Elsevier.

Holt, D.T., Armenakis, A.A., Feild, H.S., & Harris, S.G., 2007a. 'Readiness for organizational change: The systematic development of a scale'. *The Journal of Applied Behavioural Science*, 43(2): 232–255. Available at: http://jab.sagepub.com/cgi/content/abstract/43/2/232

Holt, D.T., Armenakis, A.A., Harris, S.G., & Feild, H.S., 2007b. 'Toward a comprehensive definition of readiness for change: A review of research and instrumentation'. *Research in Organizational Change and Development*, 16(1): 289–336.

Huy, Q.N., 1999. 'Emotional capability, emotional intelligence and radical change'. *Academy of Management Review*, 24(2): 325–345.

Jordan, P.J., Ashkanasy, N.M., & Hartel, C.E.J., 2002. 'Emotional intelligence as a moderator of emotional and behavioural reactions to job insecurity'. *Academy of Management Review*, 27(3): 361–372.

Kirsch, C., Chelliah, J., & Parry, W., 2012. 'The impact of cross-cultural dynamics on change management'. *Cross Cultural Management: An International Journal*, 19(2): 166–195.

Klarner, P., By, R.T., & Diefenbach, T., 2011. 'Employee emotions during organizational change: Towards a new research agenda'. *Scandinavian Journal of Management*, 27: 332–340.

Knowles, E.S., & Linn, J.A., 2004. 'The importance of resistance to persuasion'. In: Knowles, E.S., & Linn, J.A. (eds.), *Resistance and Persuasion* (pp. 3–9). Mahwah, NJ: Lawrence Erlbaum.

Martin, G.P., Weaver, S., Currie, G., Finn, R., & McDonald, R., 2012. 'Innovation sustainability in challenging health care context: Embedding clinically led change in routine practice'. *Health Service Research*, 25(4): 190–199.

National Institute for Health and Clinical Excellence, 2007. *How to Change Practice*. London: NICE.

NHS Improvement, 2011. *Overview: Change Management, the Systems and Tools for Managing Change*. Leicester: NHS Improvement.

Norshidah, N., 2012. 'The influence of emotional intelligence, leadership behaviour and organizational commitment on organizational readiness for change in higher learning institution'. *Procedia – Social and Behavioral Sciences*, 29: 129–138.

Rafferty, A.E., & Minbashian, A., 2019. 'Cognitive beliefs and positive emotions about change: Relationships with employee change readiness and change-supportive behaviors'. *Human Relations*, 72(10): 1623–1650.

Rafferty, A.E., Jimmieson, N., & Armenakis, A., 2013. 'Change readiness: A multilevel review'. *Journal of Management*, 39(1): 110–135. https://doi.org/10.1177/0149206312457417

Steigenberger, N., 2015. 'Emotion in sense making: A change management perspective'. *Journal of Organisational Change Management*, 28(3): 432–451.

Stoller, J., 2018. 'On the Paradox of "dichotomous" and "deficit-based" thinking in medicine'. *BMJ Leader*, 2: 115–117. Available at: https://bmjleader.bmj.com/content/leader/2/3/115.full.pdf

Terry, D.J., & Jimmieson, N.L., 2003. 'A stress and coping approach to organizational change: Evidence from three field studies'. *Australian Psychologist*, 38(2): 92–101.

Vakola, M., 2013. 'Multilevel readiness to organizational change: A conceptual approach'. *Journal of Change Management*, 13(1): 96–109. http://doi.org/10.1080/14697017.2013.768436

Verhaeghe, R., Vlerick, P., Gemmel, P., & Van Maele, G., 2006. 'Impact of recurrent changes in the work environment on nurses' psychological well-being and sickness absence'. *Journal of Advanced Nursing*, 56(6): 646–656.

Wanberg, C.R., & Banas, J.T., 2000. 'Predictors and outcomes of openness to changes in a reorganizing workplace'. *Journal of Applied Psychology*, 85(1): 132–142.

Weiner, B., 2009. 'A theory of organizational readiness for change'. *Implementation Science*, 4(67). Available at: https://implementationscience.biomedcentral.com/articles/10.1186/1748-5908-4-67

Wittig, C., 2012. 'Employees reaction to organizational change'. *OD Practitioner*, 44(2): 23–28.

Yongmei, L., & Perrewé, P.L., 2005. 'Another look at the role of emotion in the organizational change: A process model'. *Human Resource Management Review*, 15(4): 263–280.

7
EMOTIONAL AND COGNITIVE READINESS FOR CHANGE

New thinking

Introduction

We have argued that current change management approaches are not proving successful in managing health care changes, be this service innovation, improvement or development and that new thinking is required. We have been discussing our new thinking throughout this book, emphasising that successful change could be achieved through emotional and cognitive readiness for change which could create the energy, motivation and engagement needed for change.

In Chapter 6, we explored the concept of readiness, emotional and cognitive readiness for change, the leader's role in creating readiness for change and we introduced the AC-W model for cognitive and emotional readiness for change. We now turn to exploring and discussing the AC-W Change Management Model, its development, philosophical underpinnings and scope for managing change in healthcare and beyond.

The AC-W Change Management Model

Unlike many models that seem to ignore human emotion, this model acknowledges the role of emotions in change and the symbiotic relationship between emotion and cognition. Thus, this model could be seen as a people-centred model. People's feelings and thoughts matter in health care change because such factors could hinder or support change. The AC-W Change Management Model emerged from research within higher education (Chowthi-Williams *et al.*, 2016). Kotter's business model (Kotter, 1996; Kotter & Cohen, 2002) had been used to analyse how change was managed during the introduction of the first ever national pre-registration primary care curriculum of its kind in the UK. From the analysis a different model for change emerged, with emotion at its core. Further research using the new model

DOI: 10.4324/9781003128397-7

110 New thinking on readiness for change

during a real time change showed that emotion played a central role in change management at different levels in the organisation (Chowthi-Williams, 2018). Evidence from both these studies is discussed throughout this chapter.

The model can be conceptualised as a 'hub' and 'spokes' model (see Figure 7.1). The 'hub' being the emotional centre of the model and the 'spokes' are the necessary conditions for effective change management in healthcare. These could also be interpreted as the anchors holding organisations in place or even key competencies for the functioning of healthcare organisations. The synergy and interconnectedness between the 'hub' and 'spokes' are key to managing change with this model, allowing change agents to consider emotion throughout the change process. The model is cyclical; thus, it is non-linear, non-sequential, analytical in nature and not prescriptive. Like a bicycle wheel, the model can be manoeuvred or turned in any direction with emotion remaining at the heart of the model. Emotion, then is the philosophical foundation of the model.

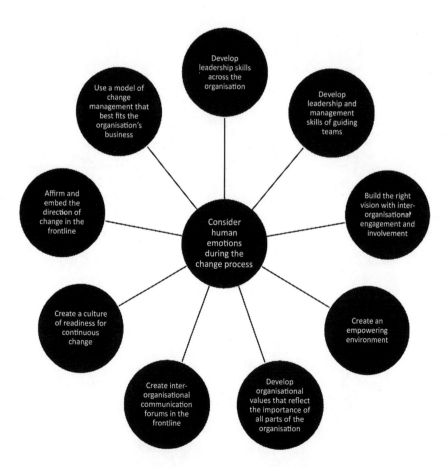

FIGURE 7.1 Diagram of the AC-W Change Management Model

As the emotional centre, the 'hub' of the model emphasises the critical role emotion plays during the change process. Change with its emotional impact can be an added burden to practitioners, which could be relieved with new ways of managing change that addresses emotions. Attention needs to focus on the emotional effects of change on health care staff, how to minimise these impacts and how to use emotion to manage change effectively. While there is evidence to suggest that change impacts people negatively, evidence within the health care setting is limited considering the extent to which change has occurred in the NHS and health care across the globe. Focusing on emotion is about recognising the important role of emotion during change. Kotter and Cohen (2002, 2012) emphasise the flow of see-feel change and believe it is more powerful than that of analysis-think change. In other words, attention to emotional reaction to change could have greater impact than attention to cognitive aspects of change, though both are needed.

The AC-W Change Management Model is adaptable and thus applicable in all health care contexts, possibly for any organisation, and for any kind of change, whether organisational or clinical, practice, small, large-scale or personal change. Within the context of healthcare, it can be used to lead service innovation, development or improvement in hospital trusts and primary care and community settings, and the various units contained within these larger organisations such as wards, teams or departments. It can be used for large-scale change such as creating new organisations be it within a hospital or primary care setting and equally, it can be applied to any type of practice change such as introducing new protocols, procedures or innovative patient services. It has a trilateral purpose: assessing emotional and cognitive readiness for change, ensuring preparedness for and the implementation of change. It allows for a bottom-up approach to change management and change leaders can choose at what point in the model to assess for emotional and cognitive readiness for change. Using their judgement, knowledge and experience of their organisation, teams, departments and workforce, change leaders can choose any of the nine spokes to begin the change process. With such valuable insight, emotional and cognitive readiness for change can be assessed prospectively, that is in preparation for proposed change; or in real time as change is occurring; or retrospectively after change has occurred. The results of the assessment of the team, wards, department, organisation or individual would then enable a preparedness and implementation plan for managing change to be put in place.

In Chapters 8 and 9, we show the model in practice. We assess the cognitive and emotional readiness for change of practitioners, managers and clinicians, based on retrospective, current and prospective change. We illustrate the model in use on its own and with Lewin and Kotter's models in organisational and practice changes as well as using it for personal change. The model is supported by a tool designed to be used for assessing emotional and cognitive readiness for change ensuring both are of equal importance and we introduced this tool in Chapter 6, providing three different versions for use in different circumstances, and outlined its role.

There may be potential criticisms of the 'hub' of the model focusing on emotion and its application though the tool considers both emotional and cognitive readiness for change. There is the danger of emotion being neglected if it is not the 'hub' of the model. For example, Kotter's research and writings could not be clearer, 'both thinking, and feelings are essential, and both are found in successful organisations, but the heart of change is in the emotions' (Kotter & Cohen, 2002, pp. 1–2). Yet his eight-step change model does not have emotion inbuilt in it. We explored Kotter's Model in Chapter 3 and note that the critics point to the neglect of emotion in his model. With most models disregarding emotion and focusing on cognition, it is important to give emotion the recognition and importance needed for effective change management. With emotion inherent in the AC-W model, it is a cue for busy change leaders to give attention to this critical aspect of human nature. Busy practitioners, teams, leaders, managers, professionals, departments and clinicians need resources that they can usefully put into practice, and this is such a resource.

The need for the AC-W Change Management Model

Traditionally, emotion has always had a bad press, currently that could not be said to be so. The pandemic has focused the spotlight on emotion and the importance of addressing it for everyone, including healthcare professionals, for whom the impact has been heavy, dealing with dying patients, colleagues, peers, their own relatives, bereaved relatives, working long hours and at the same time anxious about their own mortality. In Chapter 5, we explored the philosophy of emotion and saw that ancient philosophers viewed emotion and cognition in opposition, a struggle between heart and head and denigrated emotion as irrational. Though perspectives have shifted, it could be argued that this may not be so in regard to change management in healthcare. This negative view of emotion could be ascribed to many change approaches. Through omitting emotion in change management, there is an assumption that it should be a rational business only. However, the evidence set out in this work shows that change has major impact on people in many different ways, physically, emotionally, economically and psychologically and addressing the emotional impact of change can aid change management positively. Throughout this book, we have discussed the symbiotic relationship between emotion and cognition. In Chapter 4, we discussed sensemaking, a theory that is helpful in understanding that emotion and cognition are closely linked in responding to change. The work on emotional intelligence (discussed in Chapter 5) has enabled us to see and understand that people do not function with either emotion or cognition, but with both. In Chapter 6, we explored readiness for change and considered the original definition provided by Armenakis et al. (1993) which has been revised by Armenakis and co-authors in Holt et al. (2007a, p. 235) and defines readiness as 'the extent to which an individual or individuals are cognitively and emotionally inclined to accept, embrace, and adopt' change. We cite authors, researchers and experts whose work supports the interconnected relationship between emotion and cognition throughout this book.

Emotion and cognition are entwined and interact with each other, and this connected relationship is critical in decision making. Pessoa notes 'that complex cognitive – emotional behaviours have their basis in dynamic coalitions of networks of brain areas, none of which should be conceptualized as specifically affective or cognitive' (Pessoa, 2008, p. 148), so emotion and cognition work cooperatively rather than in isolation.

Liu *et al.* (2009, p. 4103) concluded 'that there is an interaction between cognition and emotion not only at the functional level, but also at the neurological level'. Robinson *et al.* (2013, p. 6) noted in their book that 'emotion and cognition can be distinguished but do nonetheless interact with each other in multiple ways' acknowledging the joint relationship between emotion and cognition. In the same vein, Luo and Yu (2015, p. 1039) developed a new model 'the interactive influence model of emotion and cognition' to illustrate the coalition between emotion and cognition and in particular, the extent of the interlink of emotion and reason in decision making. Dolcos *et al.* (2017) suggest there appears to be a very close relationship between emotion and cognition with emotions influencing cognition in complex ways.

This symbiotic relationship between emotion and cognition has been borne out in research on the impact of change in healthcare. Bartunek *et al.* (2006) examined effects of change and found there was both a cognitive and an emotional element to experiences of participants and Liu and Perrewé (2005) explored the role of emotion in organisational change and then developed a cognitive-emotional model of how people react to planned change, recognising this interconnection (Chapter 5).

A longitudinal study over a 12-year period explored the emotional and cognitive reactions of employees and hospital executives during organisational change (Lawrence *et al.*, 2014). It concluded that change management is not a 'rational activity' and indicated that top executives experience noteworthy emotions, the fear that they might fail, a feeling of bewilderment, distress and disorientation. There is a need to recognise that change impacts leaders too, and support and resources are needed to enable them to voice their feelings and develop coping strategies. The authors of the study suggest that 'understanding the impact of emotions can improve leadership during times of transition which translates into less resistance, quicker engagement and higher commitment' (Lawrence *et al.*, 2014, p. 257). Experiencing such emotions might encourage empathy in leaders resulting in a people-centred approach to change, acknowledging that change impacts emotions and ensuring available support and resources to ease the path of change through the organisation. Similarly, a study by Smollan (2015) within the healthcare sector showed emotional and cognitive reactions, and physical and behaviour changes during organisational changes. We discussed these in Chapter 5.

With emotion and cognition working in tandem and evidence pointing to change impacting emotion and cognition, it is crucial for change leaders to manage change in a people-centred manner instead of using a mechanistic approach. Change often fails as leaders of change do not give sufficient importance to cognitive-affective elements (Ertürk, 2008). A people-centred approach to change management means acknowledging that emotion and cognition are interdependent and an important consideration when planning and enacting change.

Emotional and cognitive readiness for change does not have a time scale in which the individual might be ready cognitively and emotionally. It cannot, as individuals will vary in their readiness and that may depend on many factors. However, through assessing emotional and cognitive readiness for change, change leaders are able to gauge the prerequisites for readiness, and put in place the necessary resources which might help speed up the process of emotional and cognitive readiness for change. The AC-W Change Management Model is underpinned with the belief that emotion and cognition are interwoven and interactive. This co-dependent relationship is necessary in managing change in health care, and this needs to be acknowledged by change leaders and thus future healthcare changes need to be managed with this underpinning philosophy.

Structure and rationale of the AC-W Change Management Model

The underpinnings of the model

There are nine 'spokes' to the model. These can be interpreted as necessary core principles, competencies or capabilities, sometimes called pillars, paths or roadmaps, of organisations, teams or departments for successful change management. The change agent can start assessing emotional and cognitive readiness for change at any point along the cycle of the 'spokes' and then put in place their preparedness and implementation plan. For example, if change leaders sense that leadership is well developed and effective in the organisation but noted that there is a lack of engagement and involvement of staff, then that could be the starting point for assessing emotional and cognitive readiness for change. Each 'spoke' is embedded with both emotion and cognition, so when assessing readiness for change, leaders are reminded of the importance and need to gauge thoughts and emotions.

The nine spokes

1 Develop leadership skills across the organisation
2 Develop leadership and management skills of guiding teams
3 Build the right vision with inter-organisational engagement and involvement
4 Create an empowering environment
5 Develop organisational values that reflect the importance of all parts of the organisation
6 Create inter-organisational communication forums in the frontline
7 Create a culture of readiness for continuous change
8 Affirm and embed the direction of change in the frontline
9 Use a model of change management that best fits the organisation's business

Spokes 1 and 2 are about development of leadership skills across the organisation including the leadership and management skills of Guiding Teams. Leadership is the most crucial 'spoke', both at the individual level and in leading Guiding Teams. In effect everyone is a leader, be it in the acute sector or primary and community care settings or in specialist care areas such as mental health, adult, child or learning disability. This may involve leading a hospital, ward or unit, a department, a health centre, a specialist unit, a sector, or as an operational manager leading many teams and services or as a senior executive, leading key areas in the organisation or as the leader of the organisation. Then there are leaders of clinical practice, professional groups, resource and finance leads, education and research leads. Guiding Teams have been identified as having a key leadership role in leading their teams through change, thus such leaders need to be the right people. By this we mean people with leadership qualities and skills, experience in managing change and have credibility amongst their peers and inside the organisation. With such expertise in mind, leaders in managing change need to build their teams, ensuring diversity and confidence in them as team leader (Kotter & Cohen, 2002).

It is effective leadership that will enable change management to be achieved. The role and quality of leadership are central to managing emotions during the change process (Fox & Amichai-Hamburger, 2001). Staff perform better when they are valued, supported, and respected, and have belief in their leaders (West *et al.*, 2011).

There has been much criticism of the leadership in healthcare organisations and its connection to poor quality of care (e.g. Francis, 2013) but the NHS has made some strides to focus on developing leadership and adopting shared leadership (e.g. NHS Leadership Model, 2013) and many healthcare curricula now have leadership development as a core theme throughout the period of education and training (e.g. NMC, 2018). Traditionally, leadership was seen as the domain of managers and staff in senior roles, but the contemporary view supports everyone in healthcare being a leader and developing their leadership and self-leadership potential. Ham (2011) puts forward that collective and distributed leadership are essential in change and should include everyone.

The style of leadership is important during change management and leaders need to be able to adopt and adapt to a variety of leadership styles and operate with emotional intelligence. In health care with its focus on people, there are many effective leadership styles and leaders need to consider the range of leadership styles in the change process and adapt their styles accordingly. Some leaders may believe it is necessary to adopt only one style throughout the change process. That is unlikely to be effective as change is a messy business, it does not always have a clear path and leaders will need to adapt their styles to deal with changing conditions, situations, environment, people's emotions, conflicts, competing priorities, culture, values, powerful and influential individuals and groups. In the emergence of the AC-W change model (retrospective study) and the subsequent research on the model in action (real time change), leadership was in action in its different forms.

In the retrospective study, the leader at the executive level was charismatic, pioneering, transformative but also took account of the situation. This could be seen through forging the first ever national change, influencing key stakeholders to come on board and continuing to drive, direct and lead people through the change. The transformational style of leadership with its high focus on people and relationships is necessary in health care where the people are its greatest asset. It's about mutual inspiration and motivation, discussion and engagement when considering prospective, retrospective or real time change. This ideally should be with everyone, especially when decision making is involved. This might be decisions about planning, preparedness or implementation of change, allowing people and leaders to be innovative and pioneering, not accepting how things are and at the same time people are able to be themselves (Burns, 1978; Bass & Avolio, 1994). This leadership approach can lead to improved performance and improved group satisfaction, compared to other forms of leadership (Choi et al., 2016) and improved wellbeing (Arnold, 2017). With health services, evidence point to this kind of leadership resulting in improved job satisfaction, a better practice environment and improved nurse retention (West, 2014).

In the real time change, there was shared leadership amongst the executive team (though there was a key leader) and they directed the course of the change. However, people wanted a consultative approach to be used through the change process suggesting a democratic, participative approach with joint discussion, ideas sought, viewed expressed and valued, and shared decision making, in effect a more democratic leadership style. Although the leadership in this change was autocratic to the extent of micro managing Guiding Teams, this kind of leadership may be necessary and can be valuable in rapid and emergency change but the workforce is more likely to accept this if the usual style is more democratic. The key is to make people feel genuinely valued and important and this approach is more likely to enhance commitment to the change.

The situational leadership style was equally of value to the executive and Guiding Team leaders. The primary care environment, the varying teams, people from a variety of different contexts, education, practice, management and stakeholders, as well as everyone's expertise and capabilities were considered. It is important to recognise that no 'one size fits all' demonstrating the need to adapt to the changing situation and changing health care environment (Hersey & Blanchard, 1969). Being emotionally intelligent may not be consistent with autocratic leadership but some leaders made efforts to become emotionally connected with the Guiding Teams. However, other leaders showed negative emotions towards other professional groups.

There is a growing body of support for leaders to adopt new ways of leading people through quality improvement, innovation and development, in effect leading change. Jabbal (2017) suggests leaders be 'enablers', thus more likely to take a people-centred approach to change management where the workforce is given autonomy, empowered and provided with support, resources, training and education to help develop their expertise, competence and confidence to manage change. West et al. (2017) note that compassionate leadership is more conducive to innovation and it is the kind of change in leadership required in healthcare. In their work, they pointed to the findings of Worline and Dutton's (2017) research with many disciplines which showed the benefits of compassion at work, that is building 'psychological safety' and being necessary for 'learning and innovation'.

These suggested leadership approaches are encouraging and open up the opportunity for current leaders to consider people-centred styles of leadership. However, with change being a constant feature of healthcare, not only is it essential to have secure leadership but these leaders need to actively involve and engage everyone in team building and promote the growth of leadership at all levels in the organisation (Erskine *et al.*, 2013). Managing change successfully does mean that leaders need to consider their style and when and how to practise their styles. They need to keep in mind that we are not all born leaders but that leadership competence, skills and qualities can be developed and take steps to be competent change leaders. Similarly, to develop leadership in all staff groups, at all levels, in all disciplines and make every effort to bridge the gap between strategic and operational parts of Trusts.

Table 7.1 summarises best practice related to spokes 1 and 2 of the AC-W model, including roles of employers and employees.

TABLE 7.1 Best practice for effective leadership in organisations at all levels, across all professionals, administrative, technical, clinical, managers and executives (self-leadership, individual, team, department, operationally, strategically)

Leader's role
- Use the tool to assess emotional and cognitive readiness for change at both the strategic and operational parts of healthcare organisations
- Make the tool available everywhere in the organisation with a drop off box available at key sites
- Leaders at all levels, in all settings and contexts to encourage its completion on a regular basis
- Leaders to collect and collate both quantitative and qualitative data from the completed tool
- Make results available: be transparent about the feelings and thoughts of staff and managers
- Set out a leadership preparedness plan for individuals, teams, professional and clinical leads departments, operational and strategic managers
- Provide mandatory leadership development programmes for all in the workforce
- Monitor leaders in their roles through feedback from peers, managers, supervisors, colleagues, teams, departments, professional and clinical leads
- Leadership competency development to become a part of the yearly appraisal for everyone

Individual's role
- Know what to expect of your leaders
- Know the different styles of leadership and how these operate
- Know your own style of leadership
- Test leadership skills of leaders through day-to-day practice
- Report ineffective leadership to the appropriate source
- Expect effective leadership from all leaders
- Assess your own leadership potential with the tool
- Set a development plan for developing your own leadership in your appraisal
- Engage in ways to develop leadership: mentor a leader/observe leadership in action in your organisation/engage in leadership programmes/practise leadership styles and seek feedback

Spokes 3–5 identify building the right vision with inter-organisational engagement and involvement; creating an empowering environment; and developing organisational values that reflect the importance of all parts of the organisation. NHS organisational structures have been shifting with changes in health care policies, be it in the acute sector, mental health, child or primary care. NHS Trusts are often managed by a Chief Executive and accountable to a Trust Board. At this level, the organisational vision and strategy are formulated, mostly without consultation with its key resources, its employees. Nevertheless, Trusts are very keen to have public involvement and engagement in developing their vision and strategies. In the retrospective change, the vision was ground-breaking and appropriate for the change that was being promoted. However, it was built and shared with senior teams across PCTs, service users, statutory bodies and other external stakeholders but frontline staff were neglected. These are the key people to involve and engage in vision building, people such as nurses, doctors, therapists, dieticians, technical staff, professional and clinical leads and many others. These are the people who will be implementing the change and thus they must be consulted.

The real time change showed there were efforts to involve people but competing priorities meant that many people could not find the time to engage in this process. However, the vision building for the change was perceived and championed as a vehicle for engagement and connection amongst the diverse professionals involved in the change. Yet it did not create an emotional connection between different groups, nor did their efforts engage and involve the full range of different professionals successfully. Again, high priority was given to involving external stakeholders, but the same effort was not given to the key people who would be delivering the change.

The challenge for many organisations is operationalising their vision and strategies and it is at this stage that change potentially fails, in particular involving and engaging frontline staff. This can be better addressed by achieving change from 'within' reflecting the need for engagement, involvement and emotional connection across the many different professional disciplines, technical and administrative staff in the organisation and with the job that they all do (West & Dawson, 2012; Ham, 2014, p. 47). Consequently, there are huge advantages to high levels of engagement, including greater happiness and better health which leads in turn to lower absenteeism and reduced staff turnover, increased patient satisfaction, positive staff experiences and reduce spend on agency staff (Powell *et al.*, 2014; Sizmur & Raleigh, 2018). It also has a cascading effect, where healthcare resources are put to use, people begin to perceive things differently and feel they can manage and cope more effectively (Ham, 2014; Dawson, 2014; Krueger & Kilham, 2007; West, 2006).

Engagement and involvement of everyone in the organisation's vision building, aiming to empower and value everyone equally within the health service, is another path to successful change. However, there has been a historic leaning towards valuing certain professional groups, such as the medical profession, and this has yet to change. Of course, it is important that the medical profession remains a powerful voice in health care decisions, but enabling the empowerment of other groups, to better represent the patient experience, will support a more workable and achievable vision. Leaders need to actively engage and involve everyone in the organisation's business, including vision creation. This is likely to lead to all levels of the workforce feeling equally valued and empowered.

Table 7.2 summarises best practice related to spokes 3–5 of the AC-W Change Management Model, for employers and employees.

TABLE 7.2 Best practice for effective engagement and involvement of people, empowerment, vision building and valuing everyone equally

Leader's role

- Use the tool to regularly assess level of engagement and involvement, empowerment, vision creation and valuing all equally
- Engage, involve and empower staff in the Trusts' vision building by giving protected time to join in vision building consultations
- Value all professional groups by ensuring they are involved in the Trust's business at all levels in the organisation, that is meetings/consultations/a place on the board/research bodies/change proposals
- Appoint involvement and engagement champions to work across professional groups/ management/settings/specialisms
- Include these values in the yearly appraisal for all in the organisation

Individual's role

- Engage and involve yourself in the Trust's vision building
- Expect good working conditions and an effective working environment
- Consult with your regulatory and/or professional bodies on poor engagement of your profession in your organisation
- Seek professional support in developing skills of engagement and involvement
- Request allocated time to attend vision building consultations
- Volunteer to be a staff engagement champion
- Encourage your peers/colleagues to engage and involve in your organisation's business
- Share the evidence with everyone on the benefits to all of engaging and involving staff in any change plans within your organisation

Creating inter-organisational communication forums in the frontline is the focus of *spoke 6*. Effective health care organisations will have channels of communication across the organisation. The strategic part of the organisation will be in communication with the operational part. However, these channels tend to be linear. Employees need a mechanism to enable them to communicate directly with the top of the organisation and vice versa. Effective communication is critical during change and in particular with the people who are implementing and affected by the change, that is those in the frontline, the practitioners and professionals.

Communication is vital for change efforts, people need to know about the change, the plans for managing it, its impacts and outcomes. Leaders need to be transparent about the change, people should be allowed to ask questions and seek assurances. Often with poor communication rumours can create greater challenges for leaders of change. People's reactions to change are influenced by emotion and cognition, communication, and involvement in decision making (Wittig, 2012).

In the retrospective and real time change, communication in a variety of forms helped not only to inform people about proposed changes, but also to engage them in the change. Face to face communication is very effective and preferred by employees, particularly at the operational level due to its emotional connection.

Canning and Found (2015) examined the effects of resistance to organisational change using a three-part methodology. Their findings suggest that a lack of communication and participant involvement during change were significant contributing factors to resistance to change and Mosadeghrad and Ansari's (2014) systematic review of the literature found a number of factors underpinning organisational change programme failure including poor communication. Consequently, change leaders need to be effective communicators during change and communicate across the organisation (Durdy & Bradshaw, 2014). A global study exploring how best to grow and maintain a culture of continuous improvement in healthcare presented ideas in the form of 'twelve foundational truths' to help healthcare leaders on this path. Communication is highlighted as key in bringing improvement thus leaders need to ensure that there is a 'common language' (Burrill et al., 2019, p. 5). With healthcare encompassing many disciplines, departments, sectors and settings, it is important for leaders to ensure everyone is given the same change message.

Health care organisations are noted for their linear communication through mechanistic methods such as reports, directives, circulars, memos, guidelines, but these ways of communicating are not always effective especially during change. Communication is much more than simply informing people about change. The message has to be grasped and understood. It takes time to process information and thus leaders will need to repeat the messages they wish to share with staff. With the challenges posed between the strategic and operational parts of the organisation communication forums in the front line involving all groups is essential in change management. Change particularly impacts the frontline and that is where the focus needs to be for leaders. With technology dominating our ways of communicating with each other, communicating during change needs face to face interaction.

Table 7.3 summarises best practice related to spoke 6 of the AC-W Change Management Model for both employers and employees.

Spoke 7 is about creating a culture of readiness for continuous change and is seen as critical for success. With constant policy initiatives, there is often little if any time to really prepare for change much less create a culture of continuous readiness for change. Such incessant change, as indicated in Chapter 1, can lead to resistance and may inhibit innovation. A culture of readiness for continuous change needs time to develop and then the challenge is for this to be the prevailing culture in the organisation, which is not easy as many subcultures exist. We explored culture in Chapter 2 as one of the many complexities in health care.

TABLE 7.3 Best practice for creating inter-organisational communication forums

Leader's role

- Use the tool to regularly assess communication at all levels and amongst all disciplines in the organization
- Create inter-professional communication forums in the frontline
- Communicate face to face with people during consultations about planning, preparation and implementation of change
- Appoint a communication champion to work across professional/management/settings/specialisms
- Include communication plan in the yearly appraisal for all in the organisation
- Engage frontline in the creating the organisation's communication strategy

Individual's role

- Use the tool to assess communication levels and approaches in your ward/department/teams/organisation
- Volunteer to be a communication champion in your organisation
- Improve your communication through observation/being mentored/training and development
- Set up communication forums if you consider there will be benefits
- Suggest ways of communicating effectively with all concerned
- Become a communication role model

However, a culture of readiness for continuous change is needed if healthcare changes are to be successful. There are no easy fixes for a culture change but lessons can be taken from evidence on how best such a culture can be achieved. In a systematic review, Braithwaite et al. (2017, p. 1) concluded that there was 'a consistently positive association held between culture and outcomes across multiple studies, settings and countries'. With culture having such an impact on outcomes, it is essential that the right conditions are in place to develop and maintain a culture of continuous readiness for change. The current challenges in health care of high emotional labour, dissatisfaction, poor engagement of staff on the part of leaders, incessant change with little visible benefit but much discomfort and pain, and poor support for staff's wellbeing, means that change leaders need to put in place resources, education, training and personalised programmes for staff that will create a culture of readiness for continuous change.

An overhaul in health care culture to create a culture of innovation and improvement is needed and could be achieved with a 'new management system', away from the kind of management style that we have been discussing throughout this book, that is from a hierarchical approach towards a more people-centred approach and to consider leadership styles, relevant technology, individual training and development needs of staff and ensuring priorities and organisational goals (Burrill et al., 2019, p. 5). Culture represents the 'thinking', 'feeling' and 'behaving' in healthcare organisations and many subculture exist (each professional group, department, ward, community and primary care, child, adult or mental health division will have their own cultures). These subcultures can be 'driving forces or may undermine quality improvement initiatives' (Mannion & Davies (2018, p. 1). It is not only important for leaders to tap into these subcultures and influence them towards a culture of readiness for continuous change but to address the barriers that such subcultures might be creating to block a culture of readiness for continuous change. Table 7.4 summarises best practice for employers and employees in relation to creating a culture of readiness for continuous change.

TABLE 7.4 Best practice for creating a culture of readiness for continuous change

Leader's role
- Use the tool to regularly assess a culture of continuous readiness for change
- Engage, involve and empower staff to develop such a culture
- Include continuous culture readiness for change as part of the organisation's vision and strategy
- Appoint champions to work across professional groups/management/settings/specialisms to promote a culture of continuous readiness for change
- Include this value in the yearly appraisal for all in the organisation
- Manage change effectively to help staff see that change can be positive

Individual's role
- Use the tool to assess a culture readiness for continuous change in your ward/department/teams/organisation(s)
- Volunteer to be a change culture champion in your organisation
- Improve your culture of readiness for continuous change through observation/being mentored/training and development
- Set up readiness for continuous change forum/s if you consider there will be benefits
- Suggest ways of effectively improving a culture of readiness for continuous with your manager/colleagues/teams
- Become a readiness for change role model

Continuous change impacts sustainability. Spoke 8 identifies the importance of affirming and embedding the direction of change in the frontline. This typically starts with the mechanism and content of communication, the rationale provided and the detail of the anticipated change. If the individual employee and the team members have been informed appropriately about the change, without the opportunity for misinformation to prevail, this same message can be used to sustain the change process. It is very important that the communication does not cease once the change has commenced. For a change to be embedded, the rationale and mechanism of the change will need to be reinforced regularly, with opportunities for employees to be supported as they face challenges with new ways of working. In this way the change can be reinforced, rather than employees reverting to older tried and tested ways of working.

In health there is a challenge in sustaining change, and it is critical to find ways to do so. Bringing about change is not easy and when change is successful, all effort should be put in to keep the change in place, but this does not always happen.

Common themes on embedding change have emerged. Involving patients and service users, staff development, support, resources and engagement were all seen as key to sustaining change. Equally important in sustaining change is board level support and leadership, with leaders becoming 'enablers' as opposed to directing change from the top (O'Sullivan et al., 2021; Jabbal et al., 2017).

Table 7.5 summarises best practice related to spoke 8.

TABLE 7.5 Best practice for affirming and embedding the direction of change in the frontline

Leader's role

- Use the tool to regularly assess whether the direction of change is being embedded in the frontline
- Engage, involve and empower staff, service users, patients and clients to maintain changes made
- Appoint champions to embed change in the frontline
- Make public the successful change and support these in the frontline
- Leaders adopt an enabling style of leadership to enable staff to sustain change
- Include this value in the yearly appraisal for all in the organisation
- Board should demonstrate their commitment to embed change

Individual's role

- Use the tool to assess whether change is embedded in your ward/department/teams/organisation(s)
- Volunteer to champion sustaining change in your organisation
- Improve your knowledge on how best to affirm and embed change through training and development
- Set up change forum/s for sustaining change if you consider there will be benefits
- Suggest ways of effectively maintaining change with your manager/colleagues/teams
- Become a role model for affirming and embedding change

The final spoke, spoke 9, concerns the use of a model of change management that best fits the organisation's business. Many organisations use the project management approach to manage change. Often a project manager is appointed to lead a particular project. This might be an individual inside the organisation but there has been a continuing trend towards commissioning external consultants. Project Management is a particular methodology which sets goals, works to time scales and outcomes and has been seen negatively. It has been seen as rather mechanistic and not conducive to engaging and involving people in planning change. While this approach is helpful in creating a project plan, the human dimension is missing.

The Project Management approach to change management could potentially be effective through initially assessing emotional and cognitive readiness for change and using the data collected and collated to set out a project plan. Leaders of change need to give careful consideration to the change approach they will use to manage change. We have discussed the lack of success of change with current approaches and thus new thinking is required on how change could potentially be managed successfully, through emotional and cognitive readiness for change, and this can be attained by using the AC-W Change Management Model to assess emotional and

TABLE 7.6 Best practice for using a Change Management Model that best fits the organisation's business for change leaders

Leader's role
- Assessing emotional and cognitive readiness for change before instigating a PM or any other change models to manage change
- PM and any change models should be used in conjunction with AC-W change model
- Have a preparedness plan to address emotional and cognitive readiness for change
- Action the preparedness plan to get people ready for any of the range of change model available
- Use the tool to regularly assess emotional and cognitive readiness for change before starting any organisational, practice or other change
- Include this value in the yearly appraisal for all in the organisation
- Leaders to promote enabling and compassionate leadership alongside the many styles of leadership
- Encourage the use of people-centred Change Management Models

Individual's role
- Use the tool to assess the change management approach best suited to your ward/department/teams/organisation
- Volunteer to be a champion in your organisation for a people-centred approach to managing change
- Improve your knowledge of change approaches through observation/being mentored/training and development
- Set up best practice change management forums if you consider there will be benefits
- Become a role model for managing change in a people-centred manner

cognitive readiness for change and implement a preparedness plan. We referred to Burrill et al. (2019) and their global study earlier. One of their 'twelve foundation truths' is a move towards 'new management systems' and here they suggest a move away from a project style approach that is based on outcomes and targets which is usually accompanied by a directive leadership style.

There is a plethora of Change Management Models, theories, improvement tools and techniques. In this book, we critique several in Chapters 3, 4 and 7. In deciding to use a model of change management, it is necessary to consider the organisation, its business, its physical resources but most crucially, its people. It is the people who lead and engage with change and it is human emotion and human cognition that require attention during change. Table 7.6 summarises best practice for use of a Change Management Model.

Summary

The AC-W Change Management Model and its application to practice emerged from research. With emotion much neglected in the vast majority of change approaches, this model gives emotion a central role in change management. Emotion is the 'hub' of the model and its nine 'spokes' are embedded with emotion.

We have outlined evidence of change and its effects on people emotionally. However, people do not function solely with either emotion or cognition but through a synergetic relationship between both. This interactive relationship is crucial for decision making. Thus, the potential path to successful change management is emotional and cognitive readiness for change through using the AC-W Change Management Model. It has a trilateral purpose: assessing emotional and cognitive readiness for change, ensuring preparedness for and the implement of change.

A tool accompanies the change model and is designed in the form of a questionnaire, to be used with the model to assess emotional and cognitive readiness for change. There may be critics of the tool, but busy practitioners should find it valuable for its ease of use and in providing them with both qualitative and quantitative data for constructing their preparedness plan.

The nine 'spokes' are integral to the model and connected to the 'hub', the emotional centre of the model. These could be interpreted as the key conditions or as anchors or even key competencies for effective change management in healthcare organisations. Each spoke is discussed and supported by evidence and complemented by best practice for change leaders and individuals.

Leadership is the most critical 'spoke' but not at the cost of any or just one style of leadership. Change leaders and Guiding Teams led by leaders need to adopt a variety of styles of leadership suited to the people they are managing; it is healthcare practitioners who will be in the thick of change both in leading it and experiencing change and thus the kind of leadership will determine whether people support the change or disengage from it. Healthcare organisations do not always value everyone in the organisation and may make people feel disempowered. Involving front line practitioners in its vision creation, communication strategy, its transformation plans and how that change will be managed will engage people in the change, create a culture of continuous readiness for change, help to embed change and generate energy for change. This energy for change can be created through emotional and cognitive readiness for change.

References

Armenakis, A.A., Harris, S.G., & Mossholder, K.W., 1993. 'Creating readiness for organizational change'. *Human Relations*, 46(6): 681–703.

Arnold, K., 2017. 'Transformational leadership and employee psychological well-being: A review and directions for future research'. *Journal of Occupational Health Psychology*, 22(3): 381–393. https://doi.org/10.1037/ocp0000062

Bartunek, J.M., Rousseau, D.M., Rudolph, J.W., & DePalma, J.A., 2006. 'On the receiving end. Sensemaking, emotion and assessments of an organizational change initiated by others'. *The Journal of Applied Behavioural Science*, 42(2): 182–206.

Bass, B., & Avolio, B., 1994. *Improving Organizational Effectiveness through Transformational Leadership*. Thousand Oaks, CA: Sage Publications.

Braithwaite, J., Herkes, J., Ludlow, K., Testa, L., & Lamprell, G., 2017. 'Association between organisational and workplace cultures, and patient outcomes: Systematic review'. BMJ Open, 2017(7): e017708. https://doi.org/10.1136/bmjopen-2017-017708. PMID:29122796

Burns, J.M., 1978. *Leadership*. New York: Harper & Row.

Burrill, G., Parker, J., & Fitzgerald, E., 2019. *Creating a Culture of Excellence: How Healthcare Leaders Can Build and Sustain a Culture of Continuous Improvement. A Global Study*. Vancouver: KPMG International Healthcare.

Canning, J., & Found, P., 2015. 'Resistance in organisational change'. *International Journal of Quality and Service Sciences*, 7(2/3): 274–295.

Choi, S.L., Goh, C.F., Adam, M.B, & Tan, O.K., 2016. 'Transformational leadership, empowerment, and job satisfaction: The mediating role of employee empowerment'. *Hum Resour Health*, 14(1): 73.

Chowthi-Williams, A., 2018. 'Evaluation of how a real time pre-registration healthcare curricula was managed through a newly designed Change Management Model: A qualitative case study'. *Nurse Education Today*, 61(2018): 242–248.

Chowthi-Williams, A., Curzio, J., & Lerman, S., 2016. 'Evaluation of how a curriculum change was managed through the application of a business change management model: A qualitative case study'. *Nurse Education Today*, 36(1): 133–138.

Dawson, J., 2014. *Staff Experience and Patient Outcomes: What Do We Know?* London: NHS Employers.

Dolcos, F., Katsumi, Y., Denkova, E., & Dolcos, S., 2017. 'Factors influencing opposing effects of emotion on cognition: A review of evidence from research on perception and memory. In: Opris, I., & Casanova, M. (eds.), *The Physics of the Mind and Brain Disorders* (Vol. 11, pp. 297–341). Cham: Springer International.

Durdy, H., & Bradshaw, T., 2014. 'The impact of organizational change in the NHS on staff and patients: A literature review with a focus on mental health'. *Mental Health Nursing*, 34(2): 16–20.

Erskine, J., Hunter, D., Small, A., Hicks, C., McGovern, T., Lugsden, E., Whitty, P., Steen, N., & Eccles, M., 2013. 'Leadership and transformational change in healthcare organisations: A qualitative analysis of the North East Transformation System'. *Health Service Management Research*, 26(1): 29–37.

Ertürk, A., 2008. 'A trust-based approach to promote employees' openness to organizational change in Turkey'. *International Journal of Manpower*, 29(5): 462–483.

Fox, S., & Amichai-Hamburger, Y., 2001. 'The power of emotional appeals in promoting organizational change programs'. *Academy of Management Executive*, 15(4): 84–93.

Francis, R., 2013. *Report of the Mid Staffordshire NHS Foundation Trust Public Inquiry*. London: The Stationery Office.

Ham, C., 2011. *The Future of Leadership and Management in the NHS: Report from The Kings Fund Commission on Leadership and Management in the NHS*. London: The King's Fund.

Ham, C., 2014. *Improving NHS Care by Engaging Staff and Devolving Decision-making. Report of the Review of Staff Engagement and Empowerment in the NHS*. London: The King's Fund.

Hersey, P., & Blanchard, K.H., 1969. *Management of Organizational Behavior: Utilizing Human Resources*. Upper Saddle River, NJ: Prentice Hall.

Holt, D.T., Armenakis, A.A., Feild, H.S., & Harris, S.G., 2007a. 'Readiness for organizational change: The systematic development of a scale'. *The Journal of Applied Behavioural Science*, 43(2): 232–255. Available at: http://jab.sagepub.com/cgi/content/abstract/43/2/232

Jabbal, J., 2017. *Embedding a Culture of Quality Improvement*. London: King's Fund. Available at: Embedding a culture of quality improvement (kingsfund.org.uk)

Kotter, J.P., 1996. *Leading Change*. Boston, MA: Harvard Business School.

Kotter, J.P., & Cohen, D.S., 2002. *The Heart of Change*. Boston, MA: Harvard Business School Press.

Kotter, J.P., & Cohen, D.S., 2012. *The Heart of Change*. Boston, MA: Harvard Business School Press.

Krueger, J., & Kilham, E., 2007. 'The innovation equation'. *Gallup Management Journal*, April.

Lawrence, E., Ruppel, C., & Tworoger, C., 2014. 'The emotions and cognitions during organisational change: The importance of emotional work for leaders'. *Journal of Organizational Culture, Communications and Conflict*, 18(1): 257–273.

Liu, Y., Fu, Q.F., & Fu, X.I. 2009. 'The interaction between cognition and emotion'. *Chinese Science Bulletin*, 54: Article 4102.

Liu, Y, & Perrewé, P.L., 2005. 'Another look at the role of emotion in the organizational change: A process model'. *Human Resource Management Review*, 15(4): 263–280.

Luo, J., & Yu, R., 2015. 'Follow the heart or the head? The interactive influence model of emotion and cognition'. *Frontiers in Psychology*, 6: 573. https://doi.org/10.3389/fpsyg.2015.00573

Mannion, R., & Davies, H., 2018. 'Understanding organisational culture for healthcare quality improvement'. *BMJ*, 28(363): k4907. https://doi.org/10.1136/bmj.k4907. PMID:30487286; PMCID:PMC6260242.

Mosadeghrad, M., & Ansarian, M., 2014. 'Why do organisational change programmes fail?'. *International Journal of Strategic Change Management*, 5(3): 189–218.

NHS Leadership Academy, 2013. *The Healthcare Leadership Model, version 1.0*. Leeds: NHS Leadership Academy. Available at: https://www.leadershipacademy.nhs.uk/wp-content/uploads/2014/10/NHSLeadership-LeadershipModel-colour.pdf

NMC, 2018. *Standards of Proficiency for Registered Nurses*. London: NMC. Available at: Standards of proficiency for registered nurses – The Nursing and Midwifery Council (nmc.org.uk)

O'Sullivan, O., Chang, N., Baker, P., & Shah, A., 2021. 'Quality improvement at East London NHS Foundation Trust: The pathway to embedding lasting change'. *International Journal of Health Governance*, 26(1): 65–72. https://doi.org/10.1108/IJHG-07-2020-0085

Pessoa, L., 2008. 'On the relationship between emotion and cognition'. *Nature Reviews: Neuroscience*, 9, 148–158.

Powell, M., Dawson, J., Topakas, A., Durose, J., & Fewtrell, C., 2014. 'Staff satisfaction and organisational performance: Evidence from a longitudinal secondary analysis of the NHS staff survey and outcome data'. *Health Services and Delivery Research*, 2(50): 1–336.

Robinson, M.D., Watkins, E.R., & Harmon-Jones, E. (2013). 'Cognition and emotion: An introduction'. In: Robinson, M.D., Watkins, E., & Harmon-Jones, E. (eds.), *Handbook of Cognition and Emotion* (pp. 3–16). New York: Guilford Press.

Siznur, S., & Raleigh, V., 2018. *The Risks to Care Quality and Staff Wellbeing of an NHS System Under Pressure*. Oxford: Picker Institute Europe.

Smollan, R., 2015. 'The personal costs of organizational change: A qualitative study'. *Public Performance & Management Review*, 39(1): 223–247. https://doi.org/10.1080/15309576.2016.1071174

West, M., & Dawson, J.F., 2012. *Employee Engagement and NHS Performance*. London: The King's Fund.

West, M., Dawson, J., Admasachew, L., & Topakas, A., 2011. *NHS Staff Management and Health Service Quality: Results from the NHS Staff Survey and Related Data*. Report to the Department of Health. London: DoH. Available at: www.dh.gov.uk/health/2011/08/nhs-staff-management/

West, M., Eckert, R., Collins, B., & Chowla, R., 2017. *Caring to Change: How Compassionate Leadership Can Stimulate Innovation in Healthcare*. London: Kings Fund.

West, R., 2006. 'The transtheoretical model of behaviour change and the scientific method'. *Addiction*, 101: 768–778.

West, S.L., 2014. *The Influence of Magnet Designation on the Recruitment and Retention of Registered Nurses in a Hospital.* Master's thesis, D'Youville College, Buffalo, NY, USA, 4 June 2014.

Wittig, C., 2012. 'Employees reaction to organizational change'. *OD Practitioner*, 44(2): 23–28.

Worline, M., & Dutton, J., 2017. *Awakening Compassion at Work: The Quiet Power that Elevates People and Organizations.* New York: McGraw-Hill Education.

8
APPLYING THE AC-W CHANGE MANAGEMENT MODEL

Assessing emotional and cognitive readiness for change

Introduction

We have covered a lot of ground. In Chapter 3, we explored a number of models, theories and improvement tools to support change and commented that although many were useful, they did not always consider the individuals involved in the change, and the way their reactions to the change could impact on effectiveness. This led us to explore additional models for change in Chapter 4, looking at those which include emotional aspects of change. We explored the nature of emotion and emotional labour, the impact of emotions and how to address emotions effectively in Chapter 5, and the concept of readiness for change in Chapter 6. So, we now have a number of models, theories and improvement tools at hand which can be useful to support readiness to change. We note that these wide-ranging models supported cognitive or emotional readiness for change but readiness for change needs to encompass both cognitive and emotional readiness simultaneously. We put the case throughout this book for emotional and cognitive readiness for change which we believe is more likely to bring about effective change in health care. This chapter provides examples of the use of a variety of real-life case studies, enabling change agents to see the importance of assessing emotional and cognitive readiness for change before attempting any change.

Using case studies, we demonstrate the potential application of the AC-W change model in creating cognitive and emotional readiness for change. In Chapter 6, this model was introduced, outlining its benefits, and in Chapter 7, a more detailed discussion on its underpinning philosophy and potential application in change management was considered. We indicated that the model provides change leaders with the opportunity to engage in the entire process of managing change,

DOI: 10.4324/9781003128397-8

that is from assessing emotional and cognitive readiness for change to preparedness and subsequent implementation of the proposed change. We discussed the critical role assessment of emotional and cognitive readiness for change plays before change can begin. To launch change without having the knowledge of people's readiness is to introduce chaos in change management. Assessment is fundamental to any subsequent change plans. We have already indicated that assessing emotional and cognitive readiness for change provides key information on the state of readiness of the organisation which then helps to put in place a preparedness plan for the change.

We use case studies in the field to illustrate the model in action. AC-W met with practitioners in the various settings to assess their emotional and cognitive readiness retrospectively, prospectively and in real time change. We present the findings and feedback for each of these. With the first case study, we used the original tool designed with the AC-W model to examine emotional and cognitive readiness for change retrospectively in a large acute hospital trust. The change involved the redesign of the current medical unit to create a new large medical division. We wanted to know people's feeling and thoughts after the change had taken place. With the second case study, a real time change was taking place and thus the tool was revised to assess emotional and cognitive readiness for this complex change involving both organisational and practice changes. For the final case study, we revised the tool again for this prospective change which we used to assess emotional and cognitive readiness for personal change of two clients through the lens of the two professionals caring for these clients.

The importance of assessment for emotional and cognitive readiness for change

We discussed the importance of emotional and cognitive readiness for change in Chapters 6 and 7 and explored the literature in this arena. Armenakis and co-authors in Holt *et al.* (2007a, p. 235) defines readiness as 'the extent to which an individual or individuals are cognitively and emotionally inclined to accept, embrace, and adopt' change. Emotional and cognitive readiness for change does not have a time scale in which the individual might be ready cognitively and emotionally. However, through assessing emotional and cognitive readiness for change and implementing a preparedness plan, individuals, teams, departments, sectors, professionals, practitioners and clinicians are more likely to be ready for change.

The theme of head and heart has been an area of discussion in the literature. We explored the debate in this arena in Chapters 5–7, and there is ample evidence that emotion and cognition are intertwined and interact with each other, impacting on us in our daily work and critical to our decision making. The assessment of emotional and cognitive readiness for change provides managers with a strategy that is relevant to their organisation, taking into account its unique features, as well as the needs of people. A strategy that is clear and decisive is likely to be more successful (Johnson *et al.*, 2011).

Developing the AC-W Change Management Model included the development of a useful tool, a simple to use questionnaire, to assess emotional and cognitive readiness (Chowthi-Williams et al., 2016). We provided this tool in Chapter 6 and discussed it at some length in Chapters 6 and 7. The AC-W model's underpinning philosophy is that emotional and cognitive readiness for change can be the key to successful change management. The questionnaire was designed to reflect this philosophy and the nine spokes of the model with emotion and cognition built into each of these. While there may be criticisms of the uncomplicated nature of the tool, we believe that it will benefit busy practitioners with many competing priorities. The role of this tool is to assess emotional and cognitive readiness for change through the collection of data from individuals about organisation and practice changes. This data can then be collated, examined and analysed. The findings and results can then help to formulate a comprehensive preparedness programme, enabling both emotional and cognitive readiness for change and an expectation of more effective and long-lasting change.

The questionnaire was used in its original format to collect retrospective data of a large-scale change in the acute care setting. It was then adapted to gather data for a real time change in Community and Primary Care, and further adapted for the prospective change involving personal change through the lens of practitioners. The participants for these case studies were all self-selected and wanted to complete the questionnaire manually. They were all employees of the health care organisations. All participants had experienced the change and were keen to share their experiences, to voice their views and opinions about the change to enable lessons for future change. Group meetings were established with participants. Data were generated from self-reporting questionnaires and informal discussions. Informal discussions were initiated by the group at the end of the group meeting. This process could be interpreted as having a therapeutic value as it gave a voice to those undergoing change in telling their stories, releasing pent up emotions, providing valuable data for future learning and not wanting an electronic record of their feedback to be traced or tracked. The case studies are detailed in the following. The first two case studies are outlined, followed by the findings from these two studies. The findings from the prospective change follow the third case study.

A case study of retrospective change: organisational change in a large acute hospital trust

It can be useful to consider a change that has already taken place, to understand how it worked, and whether there are things to learn for future changes, especially to understand the level of emotional and cognitive readiness that was or is present amongst the staff. This case study of retrospective change is summarised in Box 8.1.

The participants contributing to the exploration of the change are shown in Table 8.1.

BOX 8.1 CASE STUDY 1

Redesigning of the current medical unit to create a larger medical division

Context and background

This NHS Trust was facing a financial deficit and thus a financial recovery plan was put in place. It was a large Trust comprising of staff with a diverse range of professional and clinical backgrounds, technical, financial and support staff. It had a complicated management structure and recently there had been a re-organisation with no reduction in staff but an extension of roles for the senior management team

The assumption was that the Trust had undertaken a needs analysis using the appropriate tools to conclude that this service improvement was necessary. However, the general consensus was that the decision was purely financial as the Trust was over budget and had been so from the previous financial year.

The plan was to redesign the current medical unit with a view to improving efficiency and service delivery for patients. A plan was developed by the senior team, put forward at the Trust Board meeting and was sanctioned.

This was a large-scale change which was imposed from the top of the organisation on the workforce. The affected staff had not been consulted about this new proposal but were told by their respective managers that the change was to begin imminently. The reaction to the change had a number of serious impacts on the affected staff and their colleagues. The emotional and physical toll was high. Eventually many staff left the Trust, which led to rising costs of agency staff, high sickness rates and an unhappy workforce.

Aim of the change

Redesign of the medical unit into a medical division

Actions

- Expand the medical unit to include a number of specialist medical wards
- Close a number of hospital wards
- Merge staff across the medical unit into the new medical division
- Create a new streamlined management structure to manage this expanded unit
- Establish a smaller qualified nursing team
- Create a larger unqualified health care team
- De-establish a number of management posts
- Make the necessary redundancies in the workforce

TABLE 8.1 Participants in retrospective change case study

Number of participants	Roles of professionals
4	Newly qualified staff nurses
6	Charge nurses
3	Matrons
5	Senior staff nurses
2	Practice development nurses
2	Clinical leads – one senior clinician and 1 JR
2	Operational managers
1	Nurse leader

A case study of real time change: organisational and practice change in community and primary care

Box 8.2 summarises the case study of real time change. To explore how the change is happening in real time is of immense value, it is about getting it right as much as is possible there and then, during the change. It offers the opportunity to re-shape the change plan as the change is progressing to meet the needs of staff and patients. Staff may need additional support with managing the change, dealing with anxieties and uncertainties. Services may need to be re-evaluated based on client feedback.

BOX 8.2 CASE STUDY 2

Real time change in two organisations at the same time

Background and context

The real time change was instigated by two separate organisations. Three separate community and PCTs merged to become one large NHS Foundation Trust spanning a wide geographical area, and public health services moved into the local authority. The change was initiated by policy changes and financial constraints. It was presented to staff without consultation. These individual Trusts provided community and primary care services to the population within their geographical area. The services were provided by district nursing teams, specialist community public health practitioner teams, school nursing teams, specialist nursing teams, speech and language therapist, audiologist, palliative nursing teams, psychologists, dieticians, physiotherapists, phlebotomists and a range of other teams. This was a major organisational change which became more complex because alongside the organisational change, the Clinical Commissioning Group (CCG) simultaneously imposed practice changes on this provider organisation. The CCG proposal was to reduce hospital admissions of patients with long-term conditions and thus the management of change would now be undertaken by the community nursing service.

This very complex change was imposed from the top of the organisation on the workforce. Staff had not been consulted about this new proposal. The Trust Board had agreed the change. Not surprisingly, employees' reactions to the change were far reaching. The toll on the health and wellbeing of staff was high in particular for staff who were moving into the local authority with a new culture and new managers who had little or no experience of managing staff in health care.

A similar pattern of outcomes emerged to that of the retrospective change with additional impact on services and staff. Some health centres in community and primary care were closed, some merged, staff shifted to new locations and roles redesigned. Many community nursing staff left in the process of the change leading to rising cost of agency staff, high sickness rates amongst those who stayed and a dissatisfied workforce remained.

Aim of this change

- Create a new large NHS Foundation Trust, to span three large geographical areas, at one end was the countryside and the other included outer and inner London
- Public health services were to be moved and managed by the local authority
- Community nursing team to now set up and manage the hospital avoidance scheme of patients with LTCs

Actions

- The Trust planned to extend its services to other parts of the country, if commissioned
- Employees would be expected to work across geographical areas to cover staff shortage and sickness
- Pay scales for all staff were to be reviewed to address variations between the country areas, inner and outer London
- New management posts were to be created in line with the Trust vision

- New teams were to be formulated based on service needs
- Cost of travel of staff were to be reviewed
- Specialist nursing services would now work across all areas in the new arrangements
- A greater skill mix to be introduced in all teams

Public health proposals

- New team structures were to be developed to ensure service cover of the population
- Skill mix was to be introduced in all teams
- Teams now be managed by the LA

CCG practice proposals

- The Trust was to be monitored and reimbursed on achieving targets
- A protocol for hospital avoidance and hospital admissions was to be developed
- All patients with LTCs were to be identified and their care reviewed
- All medication to these patients was to be reviewed
- Resources currently being used by them at home were to be appraised
- New team to be formed to manage the hospital avoidance scheme

Participants in this real time change case study are shown in Table 8.2.

TABLE 8.2 Participants in real time change case study

Number of participants	Roles
6	District nurses
7	Health visitors (SCPHP)
3	School nurses
4	Primary care nurses
3	Specialist nurses/matrons
3	Managers
3	Practice development nurses
2	General practitioners
2	Primary care improvement managers

Findings from the retrospective and real time change on employee's emotional and cognitive readiness for change

A number of strong themes emerged on assessing the emotional and cognitive readiness of staff who, in the retrospective change, had gone through the change and in the real time change were experiencing the change in the present moment. While the retrospective change encompassed organisational change, the real time change included both organisational and practice changes.

The major themes that emerged for both changes were that there was:

- a lack of consideration of human emotion
- poor leadership
- inadequate communication with frontline employees
- poor engagement, involvement and empowerment of individuals and teams

The minor themes that arose were that there was:

- a poor culture of continuous readiness for change
- scant attention to embedding change
- and the vast array of Change Management Models and literature to help manage change were not used

There were some differences that were unique to the different settings and the professionals who practise in these. Where these differences have arisen, they have been highlighted.

The Retrospective Tool and Real Time Tool from which data were drawn, including the questions posed to participants in this study during the change process, are in Chapter 6.

Human emotion

The overriding theme during these organisational and practice changes was the lack of consideration of human emotion. The change overwhelmingly produced negative emotions both in the acute sector and community and primary care.

The range and intensity of negative emotions experienced included: strong anger; disbelief; frustration; resignation; longing for the familiar; a deep sense of loss. The initial reactions to the change were intense in both settings. With progression of the change, feelings and thoughts swung from intense to a feeling of resignation. This continued through the different stages of the change. There was then a constant longing for the familiar, giving rise to a deep sense of loss of colleagues, of teams, of friends and of the job as it had been. This deep sense of loss prevailed and was still present 9 months following the change.

These constant negative feelings left individuals feeling debilitated and de-motivated with little energy and enthusiasm for their work. The change had further impacted individuals' health and wellbeing, and their personal and professional plans. Eventually, these feelings and thoughts led to a sense of being 'burned out'. Many individuals either took sick leave, or started job hunting, or actually left employment and some joined job agencies.

While both groups experienced similar emotions, the sources of these negative emotions were different between the acute health care sector and community and primary care. In the acute sector, the sources of these emotional reactions were ineffective general management, poor nursing leadership, and the burden of emotional labour. Within the acute sector, individuals felt the culture of general management had always been to ignore clinical staff at the frontline. Individuals thought that most managers were poorly skilled managers, seemed rigid, structured and slightly robotic and lacked the ability to recognise the emotional toll of being a practitioner. There was disappointment in the nursing leadership. They equally were perceived as showing poor leadership at a time when the greatest impact of the change was on practitioners and patient care. Many individuals were having to work across newly created wards, loosing qualified colleagues and some of their roles taken over by unqualified staff. They felt that patient care was impacted, and nursing leadership should have been at the forefront supporting quality patient care.

In community and primary care settings, the sources of these emotions were firstly due to the heavy load of change. Three major large-scale changes were occurring at once: the creation of a new Trust; hospital admission avoidance for people with LTCs led by the CCGs; and the move of children's services to the local authority. The other major source of negative emotion amongst community and primary care individuals and teams was the invisibility of senior managers, loss of existing teams and the regrading of posts. Negativity over change was also linked to change of location of the team, increased workload, travelling longer distances to deliver care and new responsibilities with the CCG without shedding any current responsibilities. The sense of loss of autonomy within their professional roles and too many changes appeared to be a contributory factor as opposed to emotional labour and inadequate management which in the case of the acute sector contributed to the negative emotions on the change.

In Chapter 5, we examined some of the evidence on the impact of change on people's emotions and in Chapter 7, we discussed the AC-W Change Management Model in which emotion is the 'hub' and its underpinning philosophy. Despite the relentless change in the NHS, there has been relatively little literature on the effects of change on its workforce. However, based on the available literature on the impact of change, there is support for many of the findings expressed by staff in both the community and primary care and the acute sectors. Emotion and organisational change are interconnected, and as shown here, these changes had mainly negative effects on staff. The health care literature discussed throughout this book, and in particular in Chapters 5 and 7 on the impact of change, concurs with the emotions expressed by staff in both these large-scale changes.

The research on impact of organisational change is growing. A recent qualitative study on organisational change in a large hospital found that staff had 'negative expectations' and 'apprehension' on the change. Their anxieties and worries were heightened by feelings of being 'uninformed', 'fatigued' and understaffed. Some felt positive about the benefits to patients (Pomare et al., 2019, p. 1). Interestingly, some of these similar feelings were experienced by staff in these case studies who reported not being informed about the change, loss of teamwork and feelings of burnout. A longitudinal study involving nurses in Norway examined nurses' emotional experiences on organisational change at different intervals over the period of a year and highlighted emotions such as 'uncertainty', 'joy' and 'resignation' were expressed. 'Anxiety' and 'excitement' were reported before and 3 months after change was instituted. 'Frustration' and 'cynicism' were shown at 3 months and a year (Giaever & Smollan, 2015, p. 105). In our studies, participants experienced resignation and anxieties about the change which were similar to the feelings shown by participants in this study. One note of interest in this study was regarding the numbers of nurses that began in the study. It started with 20 and ended with 11 participants, with half either retired, on long-term sick or on maternity leave. In our studies many staff went off sick, left or joined agencies. These outcomes could be seen as a consequence of change but could be prevented with effective change management.

Leadership

A large number of responses reflected aspects of leadership and change. In general individuals reported experiences of poor leadership. Though both the acute sector and community and primary care sectors cited the same issues on leadership, there were differences on the impact of inadequate leadership between the acute sector and community and primary care.

Practitioners in all sectors identified a lack of effective leadership across their organisation. At the organisational level, all employees reported that they were aware that the CEO led the organisation, and that there was a management structure in place, however, there was no obvious leader they could identify with and relate to. Nurses were also aware of nursing leadership at the executive level but again there was no individual on a day-to-day basis that could be identified and accessed: in effect the nurse leaders were invisible. Despite the significant change, managers continued to manage in the same way that they had done before the change. At a time of such change, staff felt their leaders should be emotionally intelligent, but this was not the case. They remarked that their managers were frequently on leadership development programmes, yet they could not see the benefits of such programmes in the leadership practices of their managers.

A lack of guiding teams with leadership skills at ward, medical unit, health centre or organisational level meant that there was no leadership specific to the change. Some junior staff in both settings stated that clinical leadership was in place for them, but despite their best efforts, the clinical leadership was challenging to access. They expected clinical leadership to focus on clinical elements of their work and, at this time, they needed leadership to lead the change and support them through it.

At the medical unit level in the acute sector, employees stated that the manager of the medical unit appeared to be the obvious leader, but that this role was in fact primarily about management. In practice, this seemed to entail constant attendance at meetings, both internally and externally. Thus, the manager was often not seen for long periods of time and rarely visited the wards to engage with staff. The role did not seem to include time or ability to lead the unit. A similar situation was reported for the community and primary care sectors. To counter this, the managers reported that they did not view themselves as leaders, but as managers. They perceived their role as ensuring the smooth running of the areas under their domain and providing support and advice when necessary. Their main objective was to ensure financial costs remained in budget. At ward level in the acute sector, the charge nurses had a management and a clinical role. They saw their role as managing their staff and patient care on a day-to-day basis. Across sectors, the fire-fighting role together with constantly recruiting staff and pressure of budgeting was reported to give managers no time for a leadership role.

In the acute sector, there was a lack of consultation about the change, with little communication of the background to the change and thus feelings of uncertainty. Despite nurses being the largest group in the acute sector, there was disappointment with nursing leadership at both ward and organisational level and reports of leadership being non-existent. Individuals were sympathetic to the poor nursing leadership, they considered that this was due to nursing being undervalued in the organisation and a lack of power, engagement and involvement of nursing at all levels in the organisation. The nursing leadership which was present was described as autocratic, creating feelings of disempowerment and low morale. A distinction was made between organisational and practice change in which nurses would be expected to take a leadership role in the latter. Charge nurses were not seen as leaders of the organisational change as they had no prior knowledge of the change and were in the same position as the majority of staff. However, they felt that they should have been consulted by the executive nursing leadership and given a leadership role to support their team.

Within the context of community and primary care, individuals reported that the change was discussed with everyone and there were successive consultations but only after the decision was made by the Trust. However, many individuals chose not to attend the organisational meetings but were engaged with the practice change consultation. The individuals and teams in these contexts did not experience long-standing feelings of low morale or feelings of disempowerment. They felt able to discuss the practice changes and considered that on the whole their voices were heard, despite their suggestions not being taken on board. There was a greater sense of professional autonomy in this change.

All employees stated that an appointed leader might have helped to explain the organisation's rationale for the change and be able to acknowledge and deal with the strong feelings that emerged as a result of the change. But also, a leader might have been able to facilitate improved teamwork where it had broken down, boost morale, engage them in the change and provide support and advice as the change progressed and help them to consider their role in the changed organisation. Evidence of leadership skills in managers was lacking and this was a critical factor in the ability of staff members to cope with and manage the change at work and the consequent changes in their personal lives.

Equal importance was attached to the style and qualities of the leader. Individuals wanted consultation and discussion about the change. This would suggest that a more democratic style of leadership would have been preferred as opposed to the autocratic style of the senior management which imposed the change in the acute sector.

Much importance has been attributed to the failure of leadership in the NHS (Francis, 2013). We have outlined some of the evidence on the impact of poor leadership and the benefits of new leadership approaches throughout this book and in Chapter 7 on the AC-W Change Management Model, 'Spokes' 1 and 2.

In our studies, leadership at every level failed staff both in the acute sector and primary care. A combination of lack of care and poorly skilled leaders contributed to the anguish of change. The old way of a top-down approach creates emotional disconnect and impacts negatively on inclusiveness, engagement, empowerment, vision and readiness for change (Chowthi-Williams, 2018). Without doubt leaders need to practise emotional intelligence, be enablers, compassionate and transformative. These many qualities need to be reflected in their daily jobs as leaders. The question now for leaders is when and how this change will take place as the literature still seems to be suggesting it is not being practised by leaders.

Engagement, involvement, empowerment, vision and valuing of individuals and teams

Participants described that though their organisation had a vision on paper, it was not evident in practice, and that empowerment, engagement and involvement of individuals and teams was low. Vision formulation did not engage with or seek the opinions of practitioners. No effort was made to consult the frontline about any proposed change, and this elicited a feeling of disempowerment, disinterest and disengagement. This feeling was described strongly by all and they stated that this reflected how the negative way in which the organisation saw and valued them. There was a strong belief amongst practitioners that they should have been involved at every step in any change proposal.

In the community and primary care sector, staff described that there was a sense of empowerment in clinical practice and that they could make clinical decisions autonomously. However, for nursing, in acute, community and primary care sectors, empowerment to question change was discouraged by senior nurses. For the acute sector, respondents described poor clinical leadership at all levels in the organisation, and a lack of voice at senior level to represent them.

Throughout this book and in Chapter 7, we evidenced in 'Spokes' 3–5 vision, engagement and involvement, empowerment environment and valuing everyone in the organisation. The evidence suggests an overwhelming support for engaging and involvement of staff. Earlier studies to more recent ones consistently suggest happier staff leads to better outcomes for staff, patients and organisations (Krueger & Kilham, 2007; West & Dawson, 2012; Cornwell, 2014; Powell et al., 2014; Sizmur & Raleigh, 2018; Chowthi-Williams, 2018).

Communication

Across the acute and primary care and community sectors, all staff identified that any communication that had taken place about the change was stilted. This was not a surprise to staff, but the lack of adequate communication about the change did cause anger.

In the acute sector, all staff considered that there were no communication forums in the frontline and expected that this should have been a fundamental component of any change proposal. The imposition of change with no communication in the frontline raised strong reactions and outcomes from all individuals including disbelief and anger. The lack of a consultation paper was not a surprise to staff but there was an expectation of such a paper. They also stated their expectation of a series of meetings set up at different stages during the change. They should have had the opportunity to ask questions and elicit answers from the CEO. The frontline was considered by them as key, as all respondents identified that they would be the people most impacted by the change. When meetings were held by managers, most people were not able to attend due to inconvenient times, and when some did attempt to attend, managers were unable to answer or allay their anxieties and worries. The general lack of engagement in communication by managers throughout the change was disappointing. Any message of change from the organisation was thus ignored by the employees and a sense of resignation rather than involvement occurred.

Throughout this book and related to 'Spoke' 6, we have outlined some of the evidence on communication and change. We refer to a range of studies in Chapter 7, which note the role of communication during change. Change reaction is influenced by emotion and cognition, communication, and involvement in decision making (Wittig, 2012) and in a review of the impact of change in the NHS, Durdy and Bradshaw (2014) concluded that change leaders need effective communication during the change process. A lack of communication and participant involvement can contribute to resistance and poor communication can lead to change failure (Canning & Found, 2015; Mosadeghrad & Ansarian, 2014). Face to face communication is more valued for its emotional connection (Chowthi-Williams, 2018). The importance of 'common language' (Burrill et al., 2019) which is not only essential during change in healthcare with such a wide range of professionals, technical and administrative workforce but to prevent rumours and conflicting messages and make everyone feel equally valued.

These four major themes, about emotion, leadership, involvement and engagement and communication, provide an understanding of the main issues of importance to ensure effective change. The minor themes of the culture of continuous readiness for change; the attention paid to embedding change; and the use of Change Management Models to help manage change are now outlined.

A culture of readiness for continuous change

All respondents stated that the organisation was not ready for change. There were no processes, systems or plans in place and no one received any preparation for change. The impression was of a Trust in a constant state of unsettledness. Those staff who had been in the organisation over 10 years were surprised at this state of the organisation because the Trust had gone through many changes previously and those experiences, they believed, should have made it an expert at managing change.

In Chapter 7, 'Spoke' 7, we outlined some of the evidence on creating a culture of continuous readiness for change. A culture of readiness for continuous change is needed if healthcare changes are to be successful but this is not an easy task. Braithwaite et al. (2017, p. 1) conclude that there is 'a consistently positive association held between culture and outcomes across multiple studies, settings and countries'. However, Mannion and Davies (2018, p. 1) think subcultures (of which there are many in the NHS and healthcare) can be 'driving forces or may undermine quality improvement initiatives'. On the other hand, Burrill et al. (2019, p. 5) are suggesting an overhaul in health care culture to create a culture of innovation and improvement through 'new management systems', that is from a hierarchical approach, towards a more people-centred approach, for example the AC-W Change Management Model.

It is not only important for leaders to tap into these subcultures and influence them towards a culture of readiness for continuous change but to address the barriers that such subcultures might be creating to block a culture of readiness for continuous change, but this requires them to adopt new styles of management.

Attention to embedding change

Participants stated that the many changes that had been in place had not lasted and participants thought this might have been due to a lack of involvement of staff in consultation, and poor consultation with staff where some consultation had occurred. The lack of involvement in both planning and delivering of the change were highlighted as problematic.

In Chapter 7, 'Spoke' 8, we outlined some of the evidence on embedding the direction of change. The challenge in sustaining change is to prevent the 'Improvement evaporation effect' whereby new practices can decline over the long term (Martin et al., 2012). There are some common themes on embedding change which have been outlined and these include involving patients and service users, staff development, support, resources and engagement. However, leadership and the engagement at board level in the organisation is also necessary to sustaining change (O'Sullivan et al., 2021; Jabbal, 2017).

Making use of Change Management Models

All respondents stated that it was transparent to them that managers of change did not use any recognised approach to change management. This was despite the array of literature, support and resources provided by the NHS. This situation was unexpected because the senior team was considered to have the relevant change expertise, and there was a constant development programme in place for this team.

In Chapters 3 and 4, we explored some of the change models, theories and improvement tools and evidence, and in Chapter 7, 'Spoke' 9, we outlined the available evidence for change models best suited to organisations. There are a large number of possible models to use, using a model of change management that best fits the organisation is something the senior team can do to effect better change. We have discussed these in Chapters 3 and 4 and in Chapter 7, we discussed the AC-W Change Management Model which may potentially be the kind of approach to change management that the Burrill *et al.* (2019) global study indicates.

Strategy of preparedness for emotional and cognitive readiness for change

From the aforementioned case studies, it is clear that emotional and cognitive readiness for change must be embedded if those in the workforce are to work with the change and reinforce it. The assessment of emotional and cognitive readiness for change provides managers with a strategy that is relevant to the organisation, taking into account its unique features, the needs of people, one that is clear and decisive is likely to be more successful.

Strategy of preparedness for emotional and cognitive readiness for organisational/practice change

So, while much of the strategy for preparedness for emotional and cognitive readiness for change detailed earlier in this chapter applies, a focus on the following aspects is appropriate when considering organisational/practice change.

- Acknowledgement of the major impact of change on individual's emotions
- Give a voice to the individuals who are the people expected to bring about change
- Present change proposals that will win hearts rather than give lots of analysis, outcomes and trends
- Visibility of all leaders across the organisation is essential
- Develop self-leadership skills of all in the workforce and support and resource leaders to adopt the range of leadership styles, including leaders being enablers, compassionate, transformative, democratic and emotionally intelligent
- Ensure the visibility and easy access of any change plan for everyone
- Encourage engagement and involvement of the workforce in the change consultation, assessing their emotional and cognitive readiness for change and setting out the preparedness and implementation plan

- Encourage the empowerment of everyone in the workforce
- Establish frontline face to face communication forums across the organisation
- Provide open communication on change initiatives and give the rationale
- Ensure the change message is the same for everyone and shared regularly
- Support and resource individuals towards a culture of readiness for change
- Encourage the use of the evidence and literature on change management
- Support and resource staff to embed change

Having detailed the findings related to major change through case studies in the acute sector and community and primary care sectors, we now look at a case study of personal change.

A case study of prospective change: Personal change: Clients in community and primary care

The aim of using these client case studies (Box 8.3) was to explore the usefulness of applying the AC-W Change Management Model within a clinical context. Using the model for a prospective change through assessing emotional and cognitive readiness for change before the change takes place is ideal. Here the model has been tested with practitioners through a revised tool (provided in Chapter 6). This contrasts to the way it was tested for organisational and practice change in the aforementioned case studies.

Data collection was achieved through interviews with practitioners in the field (see Table 8.3), from their unique knowledge of their clients, from client notes and from their collaboration with a range of other professionals. With this knowledge and their professional experience, the model was put into action to assess the emotional and cognitive readiness of these clients to make personal lifestyle change.

Practitioners are in the favoured position of knowing their clients' needs, challenges and potential solutions. In the acute sector, this is from an illness/disease perspective. However, within community and primary care, practitioners tend to have a very good level of knowledge on determinants of health, inequalities and personal challenges, their clients social, physical and family environment. In effect they are in clients' homes and can see at first hand the influences and impact on

TABLE 8.3 Participants in prospective change case study

Number of participants	Roles
1	Mental Health Nurse
1	Health visitor (SCPHP)

their clients' personal and family health and wellbeing, for example their environment, risks to health and the determinants of health.

The case for further adopting this model for personal change in all settings is present. While professions are encouraged to use models to assess the holistic needs of their clients, in the acute sector, be it mental health, child or learning disability, the focus tends to be more on clinical needs, though some of the models allow for the psychosocial aspects of health. But with the acute sector care environment being illness/disease orientated, other aspects of human nature tend to be neglected, with little attention to the role played by emotions and clients' cognitive and emotional readiness for change especially with evidence pointing to the role of emotional health in patients' recovery.

Within the setting of primary care and community, the holistic needs of clients tend to focus on clinical and psychosocial, and more of an emphasis is given towards determinants of health. At the same time, these determinants of health have a huge impact on the lives of clients and may lead many to experience negative emotions, impacting on their health, wellbeing and motivation. To have a model that could potentially produce a more beneficial impact through assessing cognitive and emotional readiness for change can lead to improved lifestyles, impacting not only on individual lives but the nations' health.

There is a tendency in healthcare for professionals to not involve and engage clients in the construction of their health improvement plan, though this is changing. This model offers the opportunity to both clients and professionals towards partnership working whereby together clients and professional can create a plan for preparedness for the change. This plan will focus on elements that have not been given attention previously. For example, it is an opportunity for clients to explore personal leadership of themselves and their family. For some, a focus on wider issues impacting the health of the surrounding community might encourage leadership within that community, or greater confidence in having their voice heard. With clients taking such personal, family and community responsibility, change is more likely to succeed. Similarly, for some clients, communication may be a key factor in the success or failure of their personal change: who they communicate with, the tone or language used, the attitude of professionals, their family and community may drive or inhibit change. For other clients they may have emotional needs which may be impacting on their ability to make personal change.

Here, we have adapted the tool to be used by professionals, but it could further be adapted for clients to self-assess their own emotional and cognitive readiness for change. This will enable them to set out a more personalised preparedness plan for change, thus enabling them to take personal ownership of their change, driving and leading it at the pace that suits their emotional and cognitive needs, personal and social circumstances.

> **BOX 8.3   CASE STUDY 3**
>
> ### Client 1
>
> A mental health nurse with a caseload in community and primary care undertook a health check with a new client, a 50-year-old woman, who had recently moved into the area. The woman had a diagnosis of schizophrenia and the treatment for this mainly involved medication. The client was overweight, identified as non-compliant as regard to her medication and showed a lack of interest in her health and wellbeing. It was noted that her weight had increased substantially. The client indicated that she was aware of her weight gain and had been thinking about seeing her GP about a change in medication.
>
> ### Client 2
>
> A health visitor was making a second visit at home to a first-time young mother soon after the first developmental check at 6 weeks. Baby was healthy and well. However, the health visitor noted that the young mother and baby were not bonding well, the house was unexpectedly untidy, and mother was finding breast feeding a challenge. The mother confided in the health visitor that she was keen to continue breast feeding but found it a challenge due to a lack of support and feelings of low moods.

Findings from the prospective change on clients' emotional and cognitive readiness for change

The findings that emerged from practitioners indicated that a number of factors could promote emotional and cognitive readiness for change in the clients. These were: attention to emotions, leadership, involvement, engagement, empowerment and communication.

Attention to emotions

Although this mental health practitioner and health visitor had both only recently met their clients, they were both able to ascertain that their clients showed a longing to experience normal feelings and emotions and a desire to be able to self-regulate their emotions. They wished to be able to have emotional control over their lives/situations but tended to react to other people's responses rather than trust their own.

A range of situations triggered negative emotions for both clients. Their housing situation with a lack of space internally and an unsafe environment surrounding their homes, their personal relationships with partners, children and families and their relationship with professionals whom they felt at times did not recognise or acknowledge their needs. Both clients felt a constant emotional loss of control when dealing with day-to-day issues, chores, responsibilities and encounters.

Thus, to assist clients to make a change in their personal lives, support is required to develop emotional strength in the client. Helping clients to identify their emotions, be aware of them, and working step by step to develop emotional intelligence would enable clients to feel greater ownership of their emotions and a greater sense of control.

Leadership

In terms of leadership, clients were identified as in need of gaining skills in self-leadership as well as having appropriate leadership from practitioners. For both clients, there was a link with their emotional state and being able to practise self-leadership. They lacked motivation and interest in taking the lead, though they stated they wanted to do so. They were torn between wanting practitioners and others to take the lead but at the same time did not want to be led by others. There was a feeling too of wanting to engage with others through attending local support groups but both clients did not feel they had the confidence to lead themselves into such a situation. The question of how to effect leadership within the home setting needed to be addressed.

This highlights the need for every practitioner to be able to demonstrate leadership ability in the clinical situation. An effective leader will work collaboratively with the client in setting realistic and achievable goals, focused on the individual's need and endeavouring to ensure the client 'owns' their goals. A visual step-by-step picture of the journey to achievement of goals can be a useful reminder of the goals as well as the methods to achieve these goals.

Practitioners can encourage clients to build leadership skills, self-confidence and self-sufficiency through joining community groups, attending local training and support in further education, online support and tap into local resources provided by local charities and other community groups.

Involvement, engagement, empowerment and communication

There were a number of elements to consider, in order to enable clients to become more involved in their care, more engaged and also more empowered. These elements operated at the level of the family and their social network and within the wider community, as well as at the level of the individual.

At the individual level, neither client was empowered within their community or family due to a lack of involvement with the community and with family members. For both clients, the most disempowering relationships were those that involved dealing with not only the attitude of professionals but also services such as health care, housing, local authority, schools and others. However, they felt empowered dealing with charities and with some individual professionals.

Clients felt they preferred face to face communication rather than other forms such as emails, letters or phone conversations. This form of communicating was viewed as less formal and it was often easier to understand information. However, equally, face to face conversations could lead to conflict. For practitioners, tone of voice, language and other nonverbal signs are important when helping clients to make personal change. Avoiding being judgemental and communicating in a manner that increases motivation and self-confidence will be more beneficial to clients.

Working with the client to identify ways in which they can be more involved in decisions about their care, and more involved in the care itself, suggests a belief in the client's ability to make choices which will have a positive impact on their health. Planning small steps with the client, to achievement of health goals, and supporting them to develop confidence to carry out these steps is a skilled professional role.

Communication support was identified as important within the family and the social network, and within the wider community. Clients often did not have the right skills to communicate effectively with the wide range of encounters they have on a daily basis. Communicating with professionals tended to be more challenging in terms of the health care language, clients' literacy levels and unrealistic expectations on both sides. Often, they were aggressive, impatient and gave negative non-verbal messages.

An ability to communicate effectively is often assumed, but in practice this may not occur. Just as the practitioner must learn the skill of communicating with the client, so the client requires skills in communication as they take responsibility for their care. This may mean practical activities, such as setting out key parts of telephone conversations, to ensure successful communication. It may also mean a discussion of how to begin conversations with particular family or social group members to enable the client to take control, rather than be passive or aggressive in response.

Much of the strategy for preparedness for emotional and cognitive readiness for change detailed earlier in this chapter applies when considering personal change.

Strategy of preparedness for emotional and cognitive readiness for personal change

So, while much of the strategy for preparedness for emotional and cognitive readiness for change detailed earlier in this chapter applies, a focus on the following items is appropriate when considering personal change.

- Acknowledgement of the impact of change of lifestyle on individual's emotions
- Give a voice to the individual client making a change
- Develop and encourage self-leadership skills in the client
- Encourage clients to seek support from sources who might help address other challenges in their lives, for example housing/child care/finance
- Ensure the visibility of the plan for change, a copy kept by client
- Encourage engagement and involvement of the client in the change consultation, assessment of emotional and cognitive readiness for change and in setting out a preparedness and implementation plan

- Encourage the empowerment of the individual client in their lifestyle change
- Encourage clients to become engaged and involve in community groups where possible
- Provide open communication about the change and a rationale for the change. Increase face to face communication
- Ensure the change message of change remain the same and is shared regularly
- Support and resource the client towards a culture of readiness for change
- Encourage clients to read the evidence and literature on change of lifestyles
- Encourage and resource clients to sustain and embed change

Summary

In this chapter, we met with practitioners in the field experiencing organisation and practice change, and those involved in supporting their clients with personal change. We showed how the AC-W Change Management Model could be used in assessing cognitive and emotional readiness for change retrospectively and in real time. The model was successful in ascertaining the lack of cognitive and emotional readiness for change. A range of negative emotions were experienced by staff, their leaders were ill equipped to lead them through the change process and the organisation's leaders failed to engage, involve and empower these staff. Communication was ineffective at all levels, there was a poor culture of readiness for change, with change not generally embedded and leaders failed to use evidence to support change. The outcome of these changes had impact on individual staff, the organisation and patient services, though the latter was not tested here. Many staff left the organisation, the emotional toll was high and agency costs rose. Having a knowledge of readiness before any change begins or while the change is occurring means that support strategies could be put in place, thus preventing the negative outcomes illustrated here.

In relation to using the model for personal change, practitioners were able to capture the needs of their clients at an individual level which enabled them to make a personalised plan of care for their clients with a clear direction to their role.

We have detailed a large number of elements which may require consideration before a change can be successfully made. Spending time on assessment of cognitive and emotional readiness for change not only provides the opportunity to engage staff in the detail of change but also empowers them to take control. But to do this, leadership must be collaborative and inspire trust, so that employees will work positively to effect change.

References

Braithwaite, J., Herkes, J., Ludlow, K., Testa, L., & Lamprell, G., 2017. 'Association between organisational and workplace cultures, and patient outcomes: Systematic review'. *BMJ Open*, 2017(7): e017708. https://doi.org/10.1136/bmjopen-2017-017708. PMID:29122796

Burrill, G., Parker, J., & Fitzgerald, E., 2019. *Creating a Culture of Excellence: How Healthcare Leaders Can Build and Sustain a Culture of Continuous Improvement. A Global Study*. Vancouver: KPMG International Healthcare.

Canning, J., & Found, P., 2015. 'Resistance in organisational change'. *International Journal of Quality and Service Sciences*, 7(2/3): 274–295. ISSN 1756–669X.

Chowthi-Williams, A., 2018. 'Evaluation of how a real time pre-registration healthcare curricula was managed through a newly designed Change Management Model: A qualitative case study'. *Nurse Education Today*, 61(2018): 242–248.

Chowthi-Williams, A., Curzio, J., & Lerman, S., 2016. 'Evaluation of how a curriculum change was managed through the application of a business change management model: A qualitative case study'. *Nurse Education Today*, 36(1): 133–138.

Cornwell, J., 2014. 'Engaged, empowered staff are the key to better patient care'. *Nursing Times*, 110(14): 11.

Durdy, H., & Bradshaw, T., 2014. 'The impact of organizational change in the NHS on staff and patients: A literature review with a focus on mental health'. *Mental Health Nursing*, 34(2): 16–20.

Francis, R., 2013. *Report of the Mid Staffordshire NHS Foundation Trust Public Inquiry*. London: The Stationery Office.

Giaever, F., & Smollan, R., 2015. 'Evolving emotional experiences following organizational change: A longitudinal qualitative study'. *Qualitative Research in Organizations and Management*, 10(2): 105–123.

Holt, D.T., Armenakis, A.A., Feild, H.S., & Harris, S.G., 2007a. 'Readiness for organizational change: The systematic development of a scale'. *The Journal of Applied Behavioural Science*, 43(2): 232–255. Available at: http://jab.sagepub.com/cgi/content/abstract/43/2/232

Jabbal, J., 2017. *Embedding a Culture of Quality Improvement*. London: King's Fund. Available at: Embedding a culture of quality improvement (kingsfund.org.uk)

Johnson, G., Whittington, R., Scholes, K., Angwin, D., & Regner, P., 2011. *Exploring Strategy: Text and Cases* (11th ed.). Harlow: Pearson.

Krueger, J., & Kilham, E., 2007. 'The innovation equation'. *Gallup Management Journal*, April.

Mannion, R., & Davies, H., 2018. 'Understanding organisational culture for healthcare quality improvement'. *BMJ*, 28(363): k4907. https://doi.org/10.1136/bmj.k4907. PMID:30487286; PMCID:PMC6260242.

Martin, G.P., Weaver, S., Currie, G., Finn, R., & McDonald, R., 2012. 'Innovation sustainability in challenging health care context: Embedding clinically led change in routine practice'. *Health Service Research*, 25(4): 190–199.

Mosadeghrad, M., & Ansarian, M., 2014. 'Why do organisational change programmes fail?'. *International Journal of Strategic Change Management*, 5(3): 189–218.

O'Sullivan, O., Chang, N., Baker, P., & Shah, A., 2021. 'Quality improvement at East London NHS Foundation Trust: The pathway to embedding lasting change'. *International Journal of Health Governance*, 26(1): 65–72. https://doi.org/10.1108/IJHG-07-2020-0085

Pomare, C., Churruca, K., Long, J., Ellis, L., & Braithwaite, J., 2019. 'Organisational change in hospitals: A qualitative case-study of staff perspectives'. *BMC Health Services Research*, 19: 840. https://doi.org/10.1186/s12913-019-4704-y

Powell, M., Dawson, J., Topakas, A., Durose, J., & Fewtrell, C., 2014. 'Staff satisfaction and organisational performance: Evidence from a longitudinal secondary analysis of the NHS staff survey and outcome data'. *Health Services and Delivery Research*, 2(50): 1–336.

Sizmur, S., & Raleigh, V., 2018. *The Risks to Care Quality and Staff Wellbeing of an NHS System Under Pressure*. Oxford: Picker Institute Europe.

West, M., & Dawson, J.F., 2012. *Employee Engagement and NHS Performance*. London: The King's Fund.

Wittig, C., 2012. 'Employees reaction to organizational change'. *OD Practitioner*, 44(2): 263–280.

9
PLANNING AND IMPLEMENTING SERVICE DEVELOPMENT, IMPROVEMENT AND INNOVATION

Introduction

In previous chapters, we indicated that the AC-W change model addresses the entirety of the change process, assessing cognitive and emotional readiness for change, ensuring preparedness of people and resources and implementation of change. In Chapter 8, we met with practitioners in the acute sector, community and primary care, mental health and child health and showed how this model could be used to assess cognitive and emotional readiness for change retrospectively in a large-scale change in an acute trust and in a real time complex change involving both organisational and practice change. Prospective change was shown though the lens of practitioners who used the model for planning personal change with clients in mental health and child health services.

In this chapter, we show the AC-W model in action through the entire change process, and separately in tandem with Lewin's three-stage change model and Kotter's eight-step change model. We are keen to illustrate the full potential benefits of using this model on its own and in conjunction with other models. In Chapter 8, we saw the scale of the lack of emotional and cognitive readiness for change of staff undertaking change.

In our view, if change management is to be effective then implementation of change must follow on from preparedness for change, and that cannot happen without first assessing cognitive and emotional readiness for change. Thus, we consulted with colleagues in the case studies here to gather thoughts and feelings to aid our implementation of these service changes. The discussions and feedback led us to the view that cognitive and emotional readiness for change is critical in change management. Here it helped inform and shape the preparedness, planning and implementation of the patient innovation in primary care and community, service development in the acute sector, and the innovation in mental health. These

DOI: 10.4324/9781003128397-9

changes help us to see the complexity of the NHS, its management structure and potential management of change itself.

Case study 1 illustrates a prospective change, the implementation of an App to aid patients to self-manage their type 2 diabetes. The change involved three GP practices, district and community nursing services in the NHS Foundation Trust and three medical wards in an NHS acute Trust. The AC-W model was used to assess emotional and cognitive readiness for change, creating the preparedness plan and Lewin's three-stage Change Management Model was then used to implement the change.

Case study 2 demonstrates the use of the AC-W change model throughout the change process in the redesign of an acute medical unit into a medical division. In Chapter 8, we met with staff retrospectively and assessed their cognitive and emotional readiness for change, and were able to get a sense of the scale of lack of cognitive and emotional readiness for change. Here we show the extent of the preparedness of people and resources for that change and its implementation.

Case study 3 demonstrates a real time change to implement an innovative scheme to attract and retain mental health staff across the acute and primary care and community mental health services. The AC-W model was used to assess emotional and cognitive readiness for change, creating the preparedness plan and Kotter's eight-step change model was used to implement the change. (We use the terms project director, project manager, project team. We make a distinction between these roles and project style management which tends to be mechanistic in its approach to change management.)

Case study 1: implementation of an App to aid patients in primary care self-manage their type 2 diabetes. A prospective change

Background to the primary care change

The majority of the population in the UK receive their healthcare in primary care by GPs (which are independent businesses) and currently are commissioners of heath care for the population through the CCGs.

Each GP practice cares for a population which in the main is within a specific geographical area. This is not exclusively the case, nor is the population of any specific group or with a particular clinical need. GPs are gatekeepers to NHS services.

This proposed innovation led by GPs involved GP practices, an acute Trust and a Foundation Trust. The practices concerned provided services for a population with high numbers of people with type 2 diabetes. This public health crisis is addressed in recent government policy, thus providing the opportunity for this innovation in primary care.

Using a range of methods, tools and data, the GP practice teams in three practices undertook a needs analysis and identified a gap in service provision for this population. To bridge this gap, the implementation of an App to aid patients to self-manage their type 2 diabetes was proposed.

Development, improvement and innovation **153**

The CCG agreed to fund a pilot study for 9 months. If successful, the intention would be to spread the innovation more widely. It was anticipated that individual patients would be able to change their lifestyle through improved self-care. Changes could include healthier eating, increasing exercise levels, compliance with medication and regular health checks and monitoring for signs of complications. With these personal changes, it is expected that there will be an improved life expectancy and healthy life expectancy, reduction in A & E attendance, hospital admissions, and surgery for diabetic complications.

Lewin's three-stage model will be used to demonstrate how this innovation could be implemented involving the three GP practices, three hospital wards and the community nursing services.

Planning phase

Box 9.1 summarises the change process for this prospective change. The text following the box then provides details about the different elements of the change.

BOX 9.1 IMPLEMENTATION OF AN APP TO AID PATIENTS IN PRIMARY CARE TO SELF-MANAGE THEIR TYPE 2 DIABETES (A PROSPECTIVE CHANGE) – SUMMARY OF THE CHANGE PROCESS

- Innovation initiated by GP practice – Implementation of an App for people with type 2 diabetes
- Stakeholder consultation
- Steering Group formed
- Project Manager appointed
- Lewin's model in use
    - **Unfreezing**
        - Assess emotional and cognitive readiness for change and identify and address restraining and driving forces
        - Project Team established
    - **Movement**
        - Preparation and development of Project Team
        - Project Team implement App in PC/Community/hospital
        - Project Manager monitors and evaluates success
    - **Refreezing**
        - Adopt new ways of working
        - Reinforce change
        - Collect feedback and adjust
        - Spread innovation

Getting stakeholders on board to support the innovation through engagement and involvement is likely to include the following groups. This consultation could be led by a practice partner, for example a senior GP.

- CCGs
- GP representative
- Practice managers
- Practice nurses
- District nurses
- Specialist Diabetes Nurse in primary and community care
- Senior managers in the Foundation Trust
- Chair of the local patient diabetes group
- Community leaders
- Individual users
- Specialist Diabetes Nurse in the local hospital Trust
- App developer/company
- ICT
- Data manager for practices
- Improvement Director

A Project Steering Group should be established after the stakeholder consultation and would normally include the following people. However, the local situation might mean that additional people are included, especially where there are a number of different patient groups.

- GPs
- Practice manager
- Practice nurse
- District nurse team leader
- Senior manager in Foundation Trust
- Specialist Diabetes Nurse – Community
- Chair of local patient diabetes group
- Specialist Diabetes Nurse – Hospital Trust
- App developer/company
- ICT
- Data manager for practices
- Improvement Director

The Project Steering Group could be chaired by anyone but is likely to be by a senior GP who will be overseeing the innovation. It is likely this group will have the job of appointing a Project Manager to lead and manage this innovative pilot from its inception to its completion. It is expected too, that this group will support the Project Manager, monitor the innovation and support any alteration to the change plan. The Project Steering Group chair in turn will report progress to the CCG.

The project manager's role is to lead the implementation of the innovation. The lifecycle of this project involves initiating, planning, executing, monitoring, controlling and finally closing the project. A Change Plan should be established by the project manager and might include setting out the scope of the project, an implementation schedule, costs, communication strategy, a performance measurement plan, procurement contract, stakeholder involvement, risk management, quality assurance, the project team, including the change management strategy.

The change management strategy will adopt Lewin's Change Model: three stages: unfreezing, movement and refreezing, acknowledging Lewin's stance on group dynamics and action research.

The plan in action: stage 1 unfreezing

The project manager could begin this stage by bringing together the three practice teams, staff from the three hospital wards and district and community nurses. The purpose is to:

- Undertake an assessment of emotional and cognitive readiness for change (see Table 9.1 summarising this) using the AC-W Change Management Model.
- Identify the driving and restraining forces for the implementation of this innovation to get real time feedback on staff readiness for this change (see Figure 9.1).

TABLE 9.1 Assessment of emotional and cognitive readiness for change using AC-W Change Management Model: a summary of readiness for change for Case study 1

Leadership	Human emotion	Engagement, involvement, empowerment
– Transformational leadership at the top but mostly autocratic when dealing with staff	– Appears not to be any consideration of human emotion during the change process	– High GP engagement with CCGs and community groups
– No Guiding Teams or leadership in place	– No interest is shown in anyone's feelings	– Vision for GP practices not shared with MDT
Communication forum	– Change is perceived as stressful	– Change is often decided by senior GPs/partners and imposed on staff
– GPs and MDT communication forum in place on clinical issues only	– Poor consultation with practice staff and community nursing and other healthcare teams	– Often only GPs are perceived to be valued, other staff feel undervalued
Readiness for change		
– Poor culture of readiness for change	– Staff feel change is initiated and embedded for financial rewards and their wellbeing is unimportant	– Poor engagement and involvement of staff
Embedding change and change approach		– Lack of empowerment of practice staff
– Change is not sustained and project management style in place with a focus on targets		

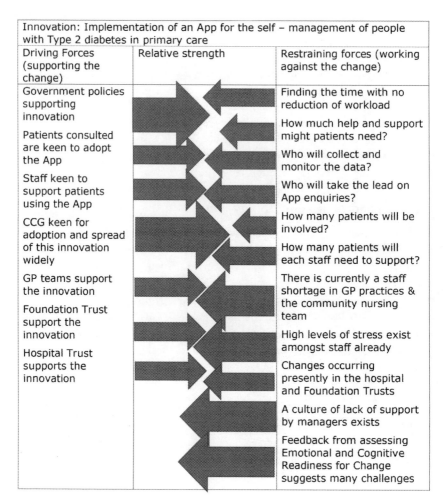

FIGURE 9.1 Driving and sustaining forces for implementation of the App

This assessment of readiness enables a better understanding of the workforce and draws from Lewin's theoretical stance on group dynamics and democracy.

Strategy for unfreezing

The aim at this stage is to get people to buy into implementing the App and form a project team who will actually implement the innovation. This takes into account the importance Lewin placed on group dynamics in successful change management. Unfreezing can be helped through establishing a series of regular meetings with staff and setting out the scope of the change, rationale and benefits, specifying the schedule and timeline, gathering thoughts and feeling about the proposed change, addressing concerns, encouraging connection with the other parts of the organisation, supporting teamwork and emphasising the need to work towards a common goal, and sharing the information with everyone.

Individuals and teams may need to be motivated to become involved in this change. This could happen through addressing the feedback from the emotional and cognitive readiness for change assessment. Using Lewin's theoretical approach, social democracy involves the workforce in the change to make it successful, including listening to concerns and suggestions for adjustments, and modifying plans to improve the likelihood of successful change. Effort will be required to encourage involvement, and negative feelings about the change must be acknowledged and considered, through wellbeing support, protected time to engage in change and personal and professional development. The project manager will need to adopt a range of leadership styles to address the feedback from the assessment on emotional and cognitive readiness (which suggested leadership was autocratic, with poor engagement and communication) and the many concerns and questions on the minds of staff gained from using Lewin's model, for example restraining and driving forces.

In Chapter 7, we discussed a range of leadership approaches and in this context the style will depend on the situation and might range from transformational, democratic, situational, compassionate or other styles. Using these different styles is more likely to encourage involvement, engagement and empowerment. At this stage, the project manager needs to be an enabler, helping people to address any negative feelings, answering the many questions posed, suggesting strategies and practical resources to support arising anxieties and stresses. The autocratic style of leadership would not be appropriate in the unfreezing phase but may be so at a later stage in this implementation.

Communication forums will need to be in place, with regular meetings between the project manager and project teams, project manager and wards, departments, primary care and community, project steering group and with individuals when necessary. It might be useful to set these up well in advance, giving everyone an opportunity to attend. The purpose of these meetings is to give a progress report on the change, identify any challenges and address these and take the opportunity in these meetings to continue to motivate staff and praise efforts.

Once the unfreezing stage is underway, a Project Team will be appointed as the group to develop expertise on using the App. Those undergoing training can then train and support patients to use it. The Project Team should include:

- Practice nurses from the three practices
- Administrative staff managing diabetic clinic
- District and community nurses in the Foundation Trust
- Diabetic specialist nurse in the local hospital Trust
- Service improvement lead
- Diabetic specialist nurse in primary care
- Senior Education Manager for the App
- Data manager and analyst for practices

Movement stage – implementation

The moving stage is the implementation stage when the change is actually taking place. A senior GP or a member of the CCG could help to support the change through his or her visibility as the change unfolds.

The Project Manager will need to action all the plan to deliver the innovation. Once the Project Team have been equipped with the relevant knowledge, skills and expertise, they can then begin the implementation of this innovation. This will include:

- Establishing regular meetings with staff in groups and individually to address emotional needs
- Establish a support network for the project team, including access to wellbeing activities, counselling and other support
- Training and development for the Project Team on how to use the App
- Setting up a support network that the Project Team can access, for example support for IT, the App itself, and administrative support
- Training and development of the Project Team around leadership skills development and patient engagement
- Designing a protocol for patient/client/user involvement
- Developing a consent protocol for all patients/clients/users
- Set up a support network and communication platform for clients/patients/users
- Designing a protocol for data collection/use of data
- Identify the number patients and which ones might be involved in this pilot
- Identifying venues for demonstrating the use of the App
- Preparing an implementation checklist (containing all actions) for staff to sign off
- Preparing a communication platform for the Project Manager to communicate with the Project Team
- Locating protected time for the Project Team to be involved in the pilot
- Locating a budget to cover staff in the Project Team
- Setting up appropriate media for spreading this innovation

These elements of implementation take account of the importance not only of the groups of staff involved, but also the groups of patients, clients or users involved.

Final stage – refreezing

At this stage, the Project Manager and Project Team must reinforce the change and the new way of working with the patients involved using the App. It is a time to ensure the pilot is working and patients are using the App effectively to manage their type 2 diabetes.

- Check with clients that they are using the App
- Get regular feedback from clients

- Remind the team of arising challenges and how to address these
- Remind people of the protocol/policies in place
- Make minor adjustments to the change based on the pilot experience if required
- Get other teams to adopt the change
- Spread change across a larger number of patients

The Project Manager will need to:

- produce a report at regular periods as agreed with the Steering Group
- monitor the project and adjust any changes
- evaluate its success across the patch
- address any arising challenges
- manage the budget and negotiate growth if need be
- support the Project Team and meet their needs

The timescales for further change implementation and the adjustments made will need to be reconsidered based on success with the change. This acknowledges the action research element of Lewin's theory. Further project reports will be needed as the implementation spreads, and these can be used to assess the success of the change and the need for adjustments to ensure continued success with the change.

Case study 2: redesign of the medical unit to create a medical division (a retrospective change)

Background to the acute Trust and change

This NHS Trust was facing a financial deficit and thus a financial recovery plan was put in place. It was a large Trust comprising staff with a diverse range of professional and clinical backgrounds, technical, financial and support staff with a complicated management structure. Recent re-organisation resulted in no reduction in staff but an extension of roles for the senior management team. The assumption was that the Trust had undertaken a needs analysis using the appropriate tools to conclude that this service improvement was necessary. However, the general consensus was that the decision was purely financial.

The plan was to redesign the medical unit with a view to improving efficiency and service delivery for patients. A plan was developed by the senior team, put forward at the Trust Board meeting and was sanctioned. In this redesign, the intention was to have a lean management team, reduce the numbers of nursing teams, extend the roles of nurses to non-nursing staff and make redundancies in the workforce.

This was a large-scale change which was imposed from the top on the workforce in a large Trust. The affected staff had not been consulted about this new proposal and employees were told by their respective managers that the change was to begin imminently. The reaction to the change had a number of serious impacts on the affected staff and their colleagues. The emotional and physical toll was high and

160 Development, improvement and innovation

eventually led to many staff leaving the Trust, rising cost of agency staff, high sickness rates and the remaining workforce in the medical division became unhappy.

The AC-W Change Management Model will be used to demonstrate how this large-scale change within this NHS Acute Hospital Trust could have potentially been managed to minimise the impacts on staff, their colleagues, the Trust and patients.

Planning phase

Box 9.2 summarises the change process for this retrospective change. The text which follows identifies specific elements of the different parts of the change process.

BOX 9.2 REDESIGN OF THE MEDICAL UNIT TO CREATE A MEDICAL DIVISION (A RETROSPECTIVE CHANGE) – SUMMARY OF THE CHANGE PROCESS

- The Trust Board initiates change: the redesign of the medical unit to create a medical division
- The CEO sets out a detailed plan at the strategic level
- A Project Director is appointed
- The CEO informs the organisation of the change
- A Project Manager is appointed at the operational level to lead the service development
- **AC-W Change Management Model in use**
  - **Assess emotional and cognitive readiness for change**
    - Leadership/engagement/involvement/human emotion/Guiding Teams/communication forums
    - CEO shares feedback and plans with staff
  - **Preparedness**
    - Project Team formed, plans for readiness for change put into action based on feedback
    - Leadership established at all levels and change reactions addressed
    - Guiding Teams (7) created to lead the elements of the redesign
    - Communication forum created and run by key leaders
  - **Implementation**
    - Phase 1 – readiness of the workforce
    - Phase 2 – readiness of medical division
    - Phase 3 – re-location of patients, staff and equipment in new division

Strategic level in the NHS Acute Hospital Trust – role of CEO

Once this change was decided by the Trust Board, the CEO should have taken the lead and set out a comprehensive plan of how to manage this change. In devising that plan the following people would have been expected to be part of the planning team. A Project Director should have been appointed to construct a plan for this large-scale change.

- Director of Medical Services
- Director of HR
- Director of Service Transformation
- Director of Medical Division
- Chief Nurse
- Director of Finance
- Director of ICT
- CCG lead
- Non-Executive Director
- Stakeholders

Strategic level in the NHS Acute Hospital Trust – role of Project Director

- Lead the change at both strategic and operational level
- Set out a project plan, including a change management strategy
- Get the plan agreed and signed off by the senior team
- Appoint a Project Manager
- Support the Project Manager throughout the change process
- Provide regular updates to the senior team

Action by CEO after change is signed off by the Board

- Announce the change to the staff affected by the service change
- Give the rationale for the change (to improve efficiency and effectiveness of services and bring about financial savings)
- Explain the nature of the change
- Give the details of what the change entails (to create a larger unit, close some existing wards, merge current staff into the new unit, create a larger, professionally unqualified health care team, create a smaller qualified nursing team, de-establish a number of management posts)
- Announce that a Project Director at the strategic level and Project Manager at the operational level have been appointed to lead this change
- Announce that the Project Director and Project Manager will be assessing emotional and cognitive readiness for change of staff
- Address any concerns expressed by staff there and then

Operational level in the NHS Acute Hospital Trust – role of Project Manager

The role of the Project Manager is to lead the implementation of the change at the frontline. They will begin by assessing emotional and cognitive readiness for change using the AC-W tool (see Table 9.2).

Redesign of the medical unit to create a new medical division

The Project Manager could have undertaken the following activities:

- Organised a large meeting with all staff affected by the redesign of the medical unit to discuss the Trust proposal and the plans
- At the ward level arranged meetings with individuals and teams, to gather views, opinions, ideas, concerns and feelings towards the change
- Met with operational managers (OP) and clinical/professional leads to get their views
- Met with change nurses/service managers/medical teams/allied health professionals and others to consider their views, ideas, feelings and opinions
- Encouraged everyone to assess their needs through the self-completed tool

With competing priorities at all levels, the shortage of time could be a factor in the Project Manager meeting with all these different staff groups to listen and hear their views, opinions and feelings and what support might be required. Some organisations might consider it appropriate to bring in an outside consultant to gather this information or for the human resources (HR) team to undertake this role, however, the workforce is likely to feel even more separated from the change and decisions about the change if external consultants or HR are used.

Following the series of meetings, the Project Manager would be expected to:

- Collate the feedback and share this information with the Project Director
- Together with the Project Director, set out a plan for addressing the needs of staff impacted by the change and establish a project plan or change the plan

After readiness for change has been assessed, a subsequent meeting will be needed, led by the CEO. The purpose of this meeting will be to:

- Listen to and acknowledge the feelings and views of the staff affected by the change
- Allow staff to express disbelief, anger and frustration
- Address low morale and discuss with staff the proposed plan to address their concerns
- Specifically acknowledge adjustments to the plan based on the assessment of readiness for change

TABLE 9.2 Assessing emotional and cognitive readiness for change: a summary of readiness for change for Case study 2

Leadership and management	Emotions	Engagement
– Poor leadership at all levels	– Appears not to be any consideration of human emotion during the change process	– Staff not engaged at any stage
– Autocratic leadership at all levels		– Nurses are not valued as professionals and have no voice at the senior level
– Ineffective general management	– Debilitated and de-motivated, emotionally unsettled workforce	
– Nursing leadership poor	– Sense of loss expressed	
– Managers continually fire-fighting and attending meetings	– Burn out evident	
	– Strong anger, disbelief and frustration	
– Invisibility of senior managers	– The burden of emotional labour is high	
– Managers display and use management skills only, not leadership skills		
– Poor clinical leadership representation at all levels in the organisations		
Guiding Teams	**Culture of readiness for change**	**Involvement**
– No guiding team to lead the change	– No preparation for change and a culture of simply imposing change	– Staff views and opinions were not sought
Communication	**Use of a change model**	**Empowerment and valuing**
– No frontline face to face communication forums	– There was a project management plan in place	– A culture of lack of empowerment exists, and valuing some professionals above others
– No communication through consultation papers		
– Message of change is ignored by employees		
– No effort to engage in communication by managers		

- Reinforce the leadership approach that will be used
- Give details of leadership at the strategic and operational level
- Remind staff of the Change Management Strategy, evidence on change management will be used to help manage this large-scale change
- Discuss the current support in place, how staff could seek support and plans for further support
- Announce the operation of an open-door policy to meet and discuss concerns and anxieties about the proposed change

- Remind staff that the leadership is an enabling one not intending to be autocratic
- Outline how future communication with staff will take place about the change
- Set out the strategy and plan for engaging, involving and empowering of individuals and teams
- Detail the approach which will be taken to creating a culture of readiness for continuous change
- Set out the plans for embedding the new change

To ensure preparedness for the change, the Project Manager will need to create a project team consisting of key people around this particular service to operationalise the change. This team will lead on the preparations needed to implement the newly redesigned unit based on the feedback from readiness for change. Through addressing the feedback from readiness, a Project Team is expected to emerge. The team would typically include:

- Clinical leads for medical services
- Professional leads for medical services
- Matrons (or equivalent) managing medical wards
- Allied professional service manager
- Operational managers managing the medical unit
- Administrative manager for medical services
- Finance manager
- ICT manager
- Head of Nursing
- HR representative
- Improvement/Transformation manager

The following issues arising from the assessment of readiness for change will require attention.

Leadership engagement, involvement and empowerment

- The Project Manager will lead and engage everyone involved by bringing together the staff and teams in the various medical wards towards the common goal of the need to improve the medical service for patients
- Feedback from the assessment for readiness will be specifically referred to, to identify the way the plans for change have been adjusted, indicating that the organisation values the experience and professionalism of its employees
- The Project Manager will lead and involve all by encouraging them to support the service improvement to see the purpose and benefits of the change, encouraging them to join forces and work together
- Guiding Teams will be generated, by setting out the preparation needed and the specific role and functions for these teams
- Create a plan for improved charge nurse leadership at ward level

- Appoint professional and clinical staff to supports staff on quality issues related to clinical and professional practice
- Assign an improvement manager to lead on addressing concerns from staff
- Engage individual staff to be self-leaders and encourage their contribution to ideas
- Approve those interested in being leader's champions for this service improvement

Human emotion

Feedback from the assessment of readiness for change suggests the staff were already unsettled prior to the announcement of this change and the current large-scale change has brought out strong emotions and a lack of belief that the change will be of benefit to them, in fact staff are already feeling a sense of loss and uncertainty about their own posts. Communication about the nature of the change is therefore vital, and individual and team meetings to address issues arising from the imposed change will be required. Some of the factors to be considered will include:

- Support in the form of one-to-one meetings with managers or team leaders to acknowledge and address feelings arising from change
- Making available resources to enable individuals, teams and groups to cope with and manage feelings through the change process, to support emotional intelligence, and to enable communication up, down and across the organisation as the change is implemented
- Provide protected time out for staff for any professional development, attending meetings, counselling, health and wellbeing sessions and any other activities needed for readiness for change
- Support phased return after sick leave
- Encourage staff to use, support and engage in and with activities through the change process
- The Trust could bring in outside support to put on activities to promote health and wellbeing
- A programme of development and support should be in place for anyone needing to re-apply for posts

Guiding teams

The Project Manager will also need to create Guiding Teams. These will be needed to lead each of the elements that will ultimately bring about the service improvement of expanding the medical unit into a medical division. The Guiding Teams are working groups. In effect each Guiding Team will be leading a mini change project to pull together all these elements for the overall service development. The Project Manager will set out the roles and responsibilities of each Guiding Team. Using these teams is an effective way of engaging and involving the staff affected by this service change. Human Resources and professional and clinical leads could provide additional support to these Guiding Teams.

Guiding Team 1

Create a patient and equipment readiness plan for the new medical division.

- Identify patients who will be moved: where they will go, when they will go, why they will be moved at that time to that place
- Prepare a plan for patients who will be discharged home or into other services
- Produce a plan (including time scale) for required equipment and safety checks

Guiding Team 2

Set out a plan for ward closure and equipment storage.

- Identify wards to be closed
- Set out time scale for closure. Prioritise these
- Establish the process of closure
- Equipment decisions: where will the equipment go? Decisions to include storage and identification of space

Guiding Team 3

Prepare a plan for merging staff across the various wards into the new medical division.

- Identify staff numbers and skill mix, that is required qualifications, experience and skills
- Set out a plan of re-location of staff, who, where, when and why
- Identify the potential for legal, professional and clinical challenges

Guiding Team 4

Create a readiness plan for the new management team.

- Set out a re-location of managers, that is who, where, when and why
- Create job descriptions
- Set out a development, support and ongoing training plan

Guiding Team 5

Outline the smaller qualified nursing team and create a preparedness plan.

- Identify the size of team and location of teams
- What will be the responsibilities of the team?
- What experience and qualifications will be needed?

- Create new job descriptions for all nursing staff posts
- Set out a development, support and ongoing training plan

Guiding Team 6

Identify the larger, professionally unqualified, health care team and their needs.

- Identify the scale of this team, number of whole-time equivalents, size and location of workforce
- What experience and qualification will be required?
- Create new job descriptions
- Set out a development, support and ongoing training plan

Guiding Team 7

Identify posts to be de-established and the process for this.

- Identify posts that are to be de-established, a time scale for this and process for informing staff
- Identify the redundancy package
- Identify the resources and support programme required for staff losing their jobs

Communication forum

The Project Manager will also need a communication forum, and this will need to be created given the lack of such a forum in the past. It needs to be a forum coordinated by the Project Manager, which meets regularly and across the organisations and at all levels of the organisation. This should be done though face-to-face meetings, emails communication, paper briefings and information on notice boards across the organisation.

The purpose of communication forum will be to:

- Update all staff on the progress of the improvement
- Identify the challenges faced and how these are dealt with
- Consider the time scale and goals and whether these are being met. Put in place plans to meet changing time scales
- Listen to anxieties and provide support
- Support progress with the schedule of change

The Project Manager will need to

- Produce a report at regular periods as agreed with the Project Director
- Monitor the project and adjust any changes

- Evaluate its success across the patch
- Address any arising challenges
- Manage the budget and negotiate growth if need be
- Support the Guiding Team and meet their needs

A range of people will need to be involved in leadership of the communication forum. For example:

- The CEO and senior team
- The Project Manager and Project Team
- Clinical and professional leads
- Human Resources
- Trade Unions
- Stakeholders

The implementation of this complex large-scale change is expected to progress through three stages. The preparation and plans led by the seven Guiding Teams will need to have been in place before implementing the three stages of this change (workforce readiness, medical division readiness, move patients), that is redesign the medical unit to create a medical division.

The project manager will need to ensure:

- Preparation of the new medical division for patients including a time scale for completion, that is the structure of medical division is ready, staff capacity and staff preparations are completed
- The hospital wards to be closed and the process for this including a plan and time scale is in place, that is wards are closed within the time scale for closure, safe equipment moved to the right location and others in storage, patients discharged into primary care and community and those to be moved to the new division are ready
- The plan for merging staff across the various wards into the new medical division is completed, that is the numbers of staff with the appropriate experience, training and expertise have been appointed, re-location agreed and all legal, professional and clinical challenges have been ironed out
- The new streamlined management structure to manage this expanded medical division is in place, that is the appropriate number of managers with the relevant experience and expertise have been appointed to new roles
- The smaller qualified nursing team is ready, that is the appropriate number of staff with the relevant training and experience to match their responsibilities have been appointed and re-location areas within the new division have been agreed
- The larger, professionally unqualified, health care team are ready, that is the relevant numbers of staff with the appropriate training and experience have been appointed and place of re-location has been agreed
- The management and other posts to be de-established has been completed, that is staff losing their jobs have been supported, given training and job searching support, counselling and the relevant redundancy package

Implementation of the change

Stage 1 – workforce in place

With the new management structure agreed and managers appointed to their positions, the next steps can begin. Staff can be appointed to their posts within the new division, for example nursing staff and the unqualified workforce. They will also need to direct the other parts of this change with the Project Manager, for example supervise the readiness of the medical division and movement of patients.

Stage 2 – medical division ready

Managers of technical, support and professional staff as well as estate managers should have a check list of all essentials that needs to be in place. This would involve ensuring all beds, resources, equipment and staff are in place ready for patient care. Equipment should have been tested for safety and documentations, medical and nursing resources all in place. Once staff and fully functioning equipment are in place, patients can begin to be moved into their individual wards within the new medical division.

Stage 3 – move patients

The transfer of patients into the new medical division could follow a plan of priority patients based on clinical needs. Discharge of those patients identified for discharge home should have been completed. Moving patients will require a large body of people to physically move patients and this plan would have been in place, ensuring patients are transferred safely to new wards.

The preceding details for the planning and implementation of such a large and complex change enable those involved in planning and implementing similar changes to give careful consideration across the range of complex issues. The negative experience of staff in this actual large-scale change showed a lack of readiness of change. Using the AC-W change model to manage this large-scale change shows the complexity of such change, and the scale of preparation required not only at the strategic level but operationally. However, the operational aspect of this change is certainly more complicated. While there is no 'one size fits all' model, the importance of readiness, both cognitive and emotional, cannot be overstated.

Case study 3: introduction of a new scheme to attract and retain staff across mental health services. A real time change

Background to the Mental Health Trust and the change

This was a large Mental Health Trust covering a wide geographical area and spanning acute and primary care and community settings. The Trust had gone through a number of re-organisations in recent times, and had been facing many challenges including high spending on agency staff. A recent CQC report put the Trust under special measures and its senior management team had been depleted since these challenges came to light, leaving the organisation's management ineffective in dealing with workforce issues.

The Trust had been experiencing staff shortages for some considerable time, well before the CQC findings. However, the senior management team consistently failed to recognise and tackle the shortages in the workforce. Exit interviews have regularly pointed to a number of factors being responsible for the challenges in attracting and retaining mental health staff both in the hospital and community and primary care settings. These included poor induction support for newly qualified and newly appointed staff, a lack of professional development opportunities and lack of protected time for development, lack of flexibility around working and a lack of compassion and care of staff. Within primary care and community settings staff expressed concerns about personal safety, large caseloads and workload together with a continued shortage of staff.

Kotter's eight-step change model was adopted, alongside the assessment of readiness using the AC-W Change Management Model, to manage this change.

Planning

Box 9.3 summarises the change process for this prospective change. The text which follows details some of these plans and their implementation.

BOX 9.3 INTRODUCTION OF A NEW SCHEME TO ATTRACT AND RETAIN STAFF ACROSS MENTAL HEALTH SERVICES (A REAL TIME CHANGE) – SUMMARY OF THE CHANGE PROCESS

- Change generated by staff and managers
- CEO sets out a detailed plan at the strategic level
- Project Director appointed
- CEO informs organisation of planned change
- Project Manager appointed at the operational level to lead the service development
- Kotter's Change Management Model in use
    - **Increase urgency**
        - Assess emotional and cognitive readiness for change with AC-W Change Management Model
        - Collect and collate data from staff exit interviews

Development, improvement and innovation **171**

- **Build a Guiding Team**
    - GT formed at strategic and operational level
    - Project Team formed
    - Working groups created (5)
    - Implementation – phase 1, 2 and 3
- **Get the vision right**
    - CEO involved and consults with staff on creating the Trust strategic plans
- **Communicate for buy in**
    - Create communication forums/regular meetings/spread message
- **Empower action**
    - Get a champion on board
- **Create short terms wins**
    - Celebrate each appointment and retention
- **Do not let up**
    - Recruit/retain staff
- **Make change stick**
    - Keep plans in place

Step 1: establish a sense of urgency

The sense of urgency could:

- Be created from the assessment of emotional and cognitive readiness for change (see Table 9.3) which would provide feedback not only on the state of the organisation but the impact on staff's emotional, mental and physical health and wellbeing.
- Have emerged from data collection of the numbers of staff leaving the organisation, those going off sick, the organisation's inability to retain staff, the cost of providing agency cover, and the cost of recruitment.
- Be shown through the voices of staff, their views and opinions about the impact the staff shortage is having their personal and professional lives, the toll on their wellbeing, increased anxieties about the quality of care to patients, risk to their registration of inadequate care and increased errors and mistakes.
- Be demonstrated from data collected and collated from users, clients and public complaints about poor quality of care.

TABLE 9.3 Assessment of emotional and cognitive readiness for change: a summary of readiness for change for Case study 3

Leadership	Need to consider human emotions during the change process	Engagement and involvement
– Poor at all levels	– Strong anger and frustration at inadequate general management, poor nursing leadership and the burden of emotional labour within mental health services	– Managers not keen to engage and involve staff in improving workforce, retention and staffing issues
– Autocratic leadership at all levels		– Senior nurses not keen on empowerment of mental health nursing staff
– Poor nursing leadership		– Staff feel undervalued and have no voice at the senior level
– Managers too busy to show leadership	– Staff emotionally exhausted	
	– Staff lacking motivation	*Culture of readiness for change*
Communication	– Staff emotionally unsettled	– No preparation for change and a culture of simply imposing change
– No frontline face to face communication forums between staff and managers	– Burn out experienced by staff	
	– Staff highly stressed	
– No effort to engage in communication by managers	– High level of anxiety and anger in the workforce	

Step 2 – build a guiding team or coalition

Once the sense of urgency has been generated, a Guiding Team will be needed, with the people who have the appropriate skills, credibility, leadership and a position of authority.

Potential Guiding Team at the strategic level:

- Director of service
- Operational managers
- Director of clinical services
- HR Director
- Director of Nursing
- Finance Director
- ICT Director
- Stakeholders

The appointed Project Director could lead this team and set out the project plan which will need to be shared with everyone.

Potential Guiding Team at the operational level:

- Clinical leads for mental health
- Professional leads for mental health
- Head of nursing for mental health
- Service managers for mental health
- HR representative

- Community mental health manager
- Community mental health matron
- User engagement manager

The Project Manager could lead the Guiding Teams at operational level and will have established a preparedness and implementation plan. At this stage, the range of issues would need to be addressed by establishing a number of working groups (Guiding Teams) each leading on a specific issue with the Guiding Team Leader coordinating the work of these groups and involving and engaging frontline staff.

Working group 1 – attrition

- Collect and collate evidence on possible causes and solutions to reducing attrition rates amongst mental health staff
- Collect data on exit interviews
- Interview current staff on their needs
- Compile a report on the reasons for high staff attrition and make recommendations for addressing this issue

Working group 2 – marketing

- Develop a marketing strategy to attract mental health staff to the Trust
- Create a plan on how to market jobs
- Identify all areas where advertising could take place
- Identify costs and benefits of different advertising strategies to attract staff
- Set out content of advertising

Working group 3 – retention

- Develop a plan to retain the workforce in mental health
- Create a Continuing Professional Development package for newly appointed staff
- Set out a career development ladder
- Identify how protected time could be located and used
- Identify mentoring and buddy support

Working group 4 – work-life balance

- Devise a plan to improve work-life balance amongst the workforce
- Explore ways of working flexibly
- Set out resources to support staff's wellbeing

Working group 5 – practice innovation

- Develop a plan to introduce innovation in practice
- Examine ways of developing practice/innovation/research in practice
- Locate champions for staff support
- Identify resources to support practice development

Once the planning is completed, implementation can begin.

- Phase 1 – advertising, interviewing and appointing staff
- Phase 2 – induct staff, ensure CPD in place, provide mentorship and wellbeing support
- Phase 3 – monitor progress of staff support and put in place plans to support staff retention, that is allocated protected time for self-development, a plan for continued professional and career development and staff engagement opportunities, mentorship for potentially new roles, ongoing wellbeing support, preparation for undertaking research, support with publication in academic journals and support any personal challenges.

Step 3 – get the vision right

The report providing data and information on reasons for the high attrition rates amongst the workforce and making recommendations should be included in the Trust's vision and mission statement. The CEO in consultation with and engagement of employees of the Trust, stakeholders and patient groups should:

- Create the vision for the Trust encompassing the wellbeing and professional needs of the workforce
- Putting them at the centre of the organisation's vision in providing quality care for patients
- Ensuring leadership at this level is enabling, transformative, compassionate, taking a democratic approach towards involving and engaging staff

Step 4 – communicate for 'buy in'

Communication will need to take a variety of forms and be led by a variety of people. A communication forum could be created and led by a range of people at different levels in the organisation to create 'buy in' to the innovation. This would include setting out dates, times and venue for communication. 'Buy in' could also take the form of regular updates via leaflets, posters, emails and communication boards on each ward, at particular sites but this must be kept updated. As examples:

- The CEO could lead at the organisation wide level and explain the innovation to stakeholders, the senior team, patient groups and staff. There needs to be discussions on the outcome of emotional and cognitive readiness for change and plans to address staff's needs. This will encourage 'buy in'.
- Clinical leads and managers could create 'buy in' at the clinical level amongst staff, explaining the purpose of the change and the expected improvements.
- Professional leads could encourage 'buy in' amongst nurses, medical and other professional groups at the operational level, team and practice level by explaining the expected positive impact on professional work.

Step 5 – empower action

The fact that the Trust has a high attrition rate of staff and the reasons are known from exit interviews, other data collected, and from assessing emotional and cognitive readiness for change should be the impetus to remove barriers.

- Have an open-door policy for staff to engage with managers at all levels
- Allow staff to voice their views on their needs and what improvements could be effective for them
- Encourage staff to identify their state of emotional and cognitive readiness for change and suggest ways to address their needs
- Find ways to encourage, empower staff and motivate staff
- Equip managers with leadership skills, emotional intelligence and resources to support staff
- Encourage professional, research and staff development forums
- Encourage self-leadership amongst all staff

Step 6 – create short-term wins

Each success of the working group should:

- Be celebrated and shared across the organisation
- Champion and spread the success at each step of the implementation
- Spread achievements on addressing staff's emotional and cognitive readiness for change

Step 7 – do not let up

In order to retain staff and ensure staff levels are appropriate:

- There will need to be regular monitoring of staff levels
- Constant feedback and action on the feedback, putting in place any new ideas generated from the feedback
- Encourage staff to regularly assess their emotional and cognitive readiness for continuous change
- Embed present change and suggest appropriate resources to continue to maintain change

Step 8 – make change stick

Managers, HR and staff will need:

- Regular interaction to ensure the plans and promises made by the Trust to retain and keep a safe level of staffing are maintained

- CEO and senior team to ensure a commitment to continue communication forums to reinforce change
- Senior managers to continue assessing emotional and cognitive readiness for change

Thus, Kotter's model, used with assessment of readiness for change from the AC-W Change Management Model, can be a useful way of planning and implementing change. The project manager will have a key role here in monitoring and ensuring each of Kotter's steps are completed, otherwise implementation is not likely. With eight steps to be implemented, the project manager may need to create a project team or appoint a deputy to help support these many steps. There will need to be a constant focus throughout these eight steps to ensure the appropriate leadership styles are used, that staff are engaged and involved at every steps in this change and that they are in a state of emotional and cognitive readiness from the inception to the completion of this change.

Summary

In this chapter, we wanted to provide the opportunity to see the model in use in a variety of settings and with different kinds of change and how change could be managed successfully. We have demonstrated the application in practice of the AC-W change model on its own and in association with Lewin's and Kotter's change models.

In Chapter 7, a more comprehensive assessment of staff's cognitive and emotional readiness for change was undertaken retrospectively, in real time and prospectively in personal change. The themes emerging there match those in this chapter. The case studies reveal themes of: poor leadership at management level; poor clinical and professional leadership; high levels of staff emotional needs but these being ignored; a lack of engagement and involvement of staff; a lack of empowerment; and the view that not all staff are valued at the same level. With change failure high at up to 70%, one might conclude that the missing link might be that staff's emotional needs are often ignored during change. The reason for these needs not being addressed is not fully researched but anecdotal evidence would point to a number of factors. We know from evidence that the emotional toll of caring is high and thus the added burden of change brings another set of emotional needs as shown in these case studies. The need to ensure cognitive and emotional readiness for change could not be more urgent, if these case studies reflect practice in other areas.

Since its inception, the NHS has undergone extensive and relentless changes. This was outlined in Chapters 1 and 2. This constant change has led to many re-organisations and reconfigurations of the structure of the NHS, not only at the top management tier but in all settings, acute, primary care and community, mental health and child settings. There is no one set organisational structure across the NHS, and increasingly with new health care policy changes, these structures have become more and more complex with many layers of management.

However, one aspect of organisational change that has remained constant is the split between the strategic and operational part of the organisation. The strategic part usually concerns itself with setting out the organisation's vision, mission statement and its strategic plans. The translation of visions, mission statements and strategic plans are undertaken by the operational element of the organisation. This complicated management structure with its many stratums of management, each with its own functions and responsibilities poses real challenges for change management. Organisations often have great change management plans, but the challenge usually is to operationalise these. It is certainly clear from these changes that any healthcare change should not to be hurried, doing so risks the many preparations either not taking place or reduced to only certain key activities.

Communication with, and listening to, the workforce is vital. Effective change management potentially requires emotional and cognitive readiness to ensure its success.

10
CONCLUSIONS

Introduction

This chapter draws together the main elements of the book. It identifies that change is a regular occurrence in any health care system, but that the way change is implemented can impact on the success of the change. Emotional and cognitive readiness for change is potentially the key to successful change management. Through assessing readiness for change, individuals will become not only engaged and involved in voicing their emotional and cognitive needs but in constructing the preparedness and implementation plan for health care change.

Having lived through many changes ourselves, studied theories of change and change management, and led change, we were keen to show through this book that change can be successful. We have pointed out many of the challenges of change in this book, and also what can go wrong to make change ineffective or unsuccessful. But we have also made recommendations for how to improve change management and we hope that both the theoretical and practical elements of this book will enable leaders of health care change to do this successfully. In this chapter, we summarise the challenges and the opportunities for change, emphasising the importance of cognitive and emotional readiness for change.

Author's perspective

The idea for this book was conceived during a period of intense and dramatic shifts in NHS healthcare policies, never experienced previously. With this and subsequent experiences of implementing policy changes in a variety of health care settings, forcing through change on senior managers, practitioners, GPs, hospital consultants, administrative and technical staff, having change imposed on us, and witnessing the impact of change on our staff's health and wellbeing without any

DOI: 10.4324/9781003128397-10

Conclusions 179

major visible benefits for patients, productivity and financial health of Trusts, and impacts on the workforce, this book came to fruition.

Change in the workplace, be it healthcare, education or business is inescapable, it is all around us as the workplace adapts to a world which is changing. In the field of healthcare, where the evidence points to the benefits of change, no one would disagree and indeed would wholeheartedly support such change. But where are these benefits? The relentless change imposed on health care, the huge number of resources given to change management, the chaos and trail of negative outcomes for its workforce, yet not seeing concrete benefits for patients, caused great concern and anxiety for us.

We felt it was our duty and moral obligation to dig deep into these issues. We examined the literature, health care policy evaluations, reports, guidelines and research studies, not only in the UK but across the globe. We talked further with colleagues in the field of health care, across a wide range of settings, across professional boundaries and at a variety of levels in acute, mental health, child and community and primary care. What is obvious to us and should be to healthcare leaders is that people achieve change, not edicts from politicians, executives, managers, tools, techniques, model or strategies, these are only resources to aid change management. Yet from our experiences and observations, people seem to be the least important element in change management. We concluded that change management in its current format in the health sector is unsustainable, and new thinking is required on managing health care changes.

In this book, we have argued for this new thinking, with the focus on human nature. We believe that the key to successful change management is cognitive and emotional readiness for change. Through research by one of the authors (AC-W), the AC-W Change Management Model was developed with people at the centre of change, health care staff from diverse backgrounds, experiences, levels, different health care settings and situations. AC-W then conducted further research to test the model and concluded that cognitive and emotional readiness for change is necessary for effective healthcare change management. With practitioners and managers in the NHS, in acute, primary care and community, mental health and child sectors, the model was put into action on a larger scale to illustrate how change had the potential to be managed effectively.

The Tony Blair government was elected in 1997 and Labour remained in power until 2010. During Blair's tenure, the government proceeded to modernise the NHS, with a shift in health care policy towards primary care. The commission of health care services for the NHS was handed to PCTs while hospitals and the private sector took on the provider role, with great excitement and motivation that at long last primary care was being given the recognition it deserved. No longer would it be the poor relation of the acute sector but it would hold great power, and with it the responsibility of modernising the NHS. AC-W joined a London Primary Care Group (PCG) in 2000. These feelings of hope and excitement were quickly dispelled when PCGs were turned into PCTs and almost everyone had to re-apply either for their own posts or for one of many newly created jobs in the new PCTs. Of course, what staff were not told was there were not enough posts for everyone.

Alongside the newly created PCTs, new services were being designed and redesigned. The PCT took over the management of failing GP practices and some acute services. Hospitals were demanding more money for the acute sector, while tending to ignore any movement of their services into primary care. New technology was being introduced widely and new GP practices and new services were being either developed or improved in both primary and secondary care. The pressure on PCTs to achieve their targets in order that they could retain their PCT's star rating was unrelenting. Not only were we experiencing change ourselves as senior managers, but having to impose change on our managers and hundreds of professionals in the frontline both in primary care and the acute sector. The change impacted staff, managers, senior managers and executives, all of whom were either agents of change or had change imposed upon them.

The impact on people and resources was far reaching. For its people, the effects were physical, emotional and psychological. The level of sickness grew, staff were highly stressed, there was a huge turnover of staff, some took early retirement for the sake of their health, many left the organisations, the size of agency staff grew (most of our budget was spent here), patients were no happier than they had been with the care they received prior to the changes. Indeed, many were disappointed as the policy shifts created expectations. PCTs and their acute sector counterparts were constantly in financial deficit, which then led to further re-organisations and staff redundancies. The scale of the pain of change was evident with staff at all levels in the NHS, from frontline staff to CEOs.

Thinking that such mayhem was the domain of healthcare, a move was made into the world of academia. The theme of change was equally relentless in higher education (HE). There were continued mergers of schools, departments, teams, education services, ICT, student services and others. There were new curricula changes, changes in healthcare and education practice, teaching and learning approaches, technology, the creation of hybrid roles, newly added responsibilities for academics, change in assessments and student experience, and regulatory changes for health care professionals and others. Alongside this, the structural changes in the NHS often meant that we had to change who we related to in the health service to continue to achieve the same outcome.

Our connection with the NHS continued through maintaining our own clinical practice, supporting healthcare students in their clinical practice, and engaging in service improvement, innovation and development with our NHS colleagues. It became evident that our earlier experiences of health care policy changes and how these were managed in the NHS was not unique to the Tony Blair government. Health care policy changes continued unrelentingly with even more serious impact on healthcare and its people, who care for the nation's health.

The Health and Social Care Act of 2012, under the coalition Conservative/Liberal Democrat government, dominated the first part of the second decade of the new millennium. It caused considerable damage, with more re-organisation, complexity and confusion. Also at this time, the Francis Inquiry Report was published, highlighting the dreadful standards of care within a system which did not prioritise the care of patients and did not encourage staff to challenge poor standards. The culture was not conducive to good care, there was a need for honesty, for openness and for effective leadership.

But lessons about change have not been learned. Just when the NHS has proven its worth with the current pandemic, a new set of proposed changes were announced in 2021 for NHS England without regard to reasons for previous failures. Described by the Nuffield Trust (2021, p. 1) as 'the biggest legislative overhaul of the NHS presented to the House of Commons for a decade', the Health and Care Bill 2021 brings structural reform. The current CCGs across the country will be replaced by integrated care systems (ICS) with the task of bringing all systems together to plan care, but without much needed local scrutiny. The proposed new groupings are larger than the current ones, so that allocation of funds might be less specific to areas of need. The Government will give itself new powers to direct the NHS in England and involve themselves in local changes, with the potential that even small changes will need government approval. There is concern that ministers will have the power to intervene in decisions currently made by experienced health professionals.

The internal market will remain but instead of competition there should be collaboration. While this is to be welcomed, stagnation could occur where co-operation is lacking. Part of this collaboration is reflected in the expectation of better co-operation between the NHS and social care. However, the current crisis in social care, which has been worsening, is not addressed by the Bill.

The case for current change management failure

The pace of change, role of national bodies and lack of data on change success/failure

The health policy initiatives by successive governments have been relentless. Even in the current pandemic crisis, new policy changes have been announced. The timeline of these policies issued by governments shows the sheer scale and volume of these, not to mention the complexities of the changes set out in them. The speed at which these have emerged time and time again makes it near impossible for busy practitioners, whose core role is to care, to find the time to read and digest these, much less lead or involve themselves in these changes.

Various UK governments established a number of improvement agencies, supported by staff, brought in external consultants and established financial remuneration for successful improvements in health care. These bodies have produced and promoted improvement guides, a diverse range of models, approaches, tools and an array of training and development programmes.

We wanted to know how these healthcare policy changes are being managed in the NHS and the rate of success and failure. However, there is little or no data available on the percentage rates of success or failure of policy changes nor is it clear how change is managed in individual Trusts, regionally or nationally in the NHS or in the countries in the UK. We were unable to ascertain whether managers, leaders or change agents in Trusts were using specific Change Management Models, theories, tools or strategies for specific kinds of change, if so, what were these and which ones were effective? We wanted to know too whether the literature is consulted on how best to manage change.

In effect there is no unified view on how best to manage change, which approach is best, or how change agents would arrive at decisions regarding which approach to use to implement their change. It could be argued that having a unified voice may not be helpful because change has to consider context, settings, people and costs, but clearer and more specific guidance to support leaders of change across a range of contexts would be useful.

The question needs to be asked, why have these national bodies and the vast resources allocated to them been created if they cannot give a clear steer or consensus on how best to manage change and point out rates of successes and failures? Furthermore, how can change be managed effectively if the resources to support us are constantly themselves going through change. It is ironic that while these agencies are busy telling us to manage change, they themselves are at the mercy of change.

The absence of benefit

It seems logical if governments are making changes to health care and justifying these on the grounds of benefits for patients and the NHS, then there should be improvements in the nations' health, the health of NHS finances and a healthy and happy workforce. In examining the literature, various health care policy evaluations, reports and research, we found that while there have been some benefits for patients, these have generally been short lived. There have been occasional notable exceptions, such as the improvements in cardiac health from the legislation banning cigarette smoking in public places. But overwhelmingly, despite the policy changes, the huge volume of resources spent on change management and claims that policy changes will improve the quality of health of the population, this has not happened, rather, mortality and morbidity are worsening. Inequalities have grown between those who have and those who do not.

Evidence shows the differences in health outcomes and healthy life expectancy across the four UK countries and internationally with countries of similar wealth. Socio-economic status plays a key role in life expectancy and healthy life expectancy. People from higher socio-economic background and those who live in the south of the country have better health outcomes than those who live in deprived areas and in other parts of the UK. Scotland has lower life expectancy for both males and females compared to the other countries that make up the UK. Infant mortality has increased in deprived areas and a 'death of despair' in the population aged 45–54 in present in the country, where people are dying from drug and alcohol over consumption, suicides and alcohol-related diseases. We are a wealthy country but international comparison shows male and female life expectancy across all UK countries to be below that of their counterparts in the EU.

How to finance the NHS has created many a debate amongst politicians, the public, media and professional and regulatory bodies. Governments have attempted to address the financing of the NHS though means of policy changes. Through change often the expectation is that money will be saved, and productivity increased. However, people are waiting longer than 18 weeks for hospital treatment and 2.5 million patients had to wait longer than the target of 4 hours in A & E. Financially Trusts and CCGs are in poor health. Many are expected to overspend by half their budget, CCGs' financial positions are precarious with the possibility of their overspending addressed either by deferring or annulling their accounts. The promise of 5000 more GPs has not been forthcoming instead there is a reduction. The number of people being referred to psychological therapies has reduced and the plan for digital health records is not likely to meet its deadline, with the nations' health showing differences across socio-economic groups, the four countries of the UK and internationally, and no increase in productivity. Why then do these incessant policy changes continue?

Working in health is having a toll on the wellbeing of the workforce. Currently, there is a huge shortage of staff and many continue to leave the profession. It is not a surprise to find evidence of a link between staff engagement, satisfaction and patient outcomes, safety, quality of care and health. This is not just the case in the UK but across the globe where studies point to the association between staff engagement, satisfaction and patient outcomes.

There is a continued feeling of dissatisfaction amongst many staff, be they doctors, nurses or other professional groups. In particular for nursing, evidence of compassion fatigue, burnout and secondary trauma were connected to their dissatisfaction. The source of these feelings is linked to high patient volumes, caring for patients with complex health needs, high workload, ethical dilemmas and conflicting values between patients and those who care for them. Happy staff are linked to better health outcomes for patients and that requires their engagement and involvement in all levels in the organisation.

Complexity and the NHS

Through our many years of experience in the NHS, we encountered its complexities. The complicated nature of the NHS has multiplied with even more changes imposed on it. The latest video compiled by the Kings Fund brings home its many complexities, particularly the complexity of NHS England. The current approach to change tends to be hierarchical, disregarding the input of knowledgeable professionals with their understanding of the ethical dilemmas faced, the complexities of patient care and the local culture. This valuable resource is often overlooked when it comes to planning and implementing change.

If change management is to be effective, the layers of management within organisations needs consideration, thereby lessening the hierarchical division at all levels and especially between the strategic and operational parts of the organisation, giving more importance to the operations, strengthening the leadership and apportioning more resources. Professionals have to practise in accordance with their respective codes and instead of employers questioning these values, staff should be supported and encouraged through interprofessional working, recognising the ethical and moral dilemmas faced every day. It is important that leaders of Trusts acknowledge that caring is not a business for those who care for the nation but a duty, a moral imperative, a vocation and thus staff need acknowledgement, support and resources to address the many dilemmas they will encounter as they deliver health care.

Since devolution of health care, the different nations of the UK have evolved separately, creating another layer of complexity. Opportunities to collect data to consider which policies work best have been missed. Comparable data are lacking, so that changes made cannot be judged to determine success.

Politicians' involvement in the NHS has caused chaotic intervention at the operational level. Politics is best removed from the day-to-day operation of the service. Why appoint people with experience and skills to take charge of Trusts, if politicians are then going to tell them how to run these. Recent announcements on more policy changes in the midst of a pandemic suggest that lessons have not been learned about this interference in operational aspects of the health service. Politicians do need to find a way of working with the management of the NHS that will bring cohesiveness instead of causing chaos.

Poor attention to human nature in current change approaches

There is a gamut of change approaches, models and theories of change with differing and diverse philosophies. These could easily confuse people when deciding which approach might work best, whether to use the planned or emergent approach or something that sits in between these two. In 2001, the NHS drew together all existing change strategies, models and approaches across the globe in an effort to support practitioners implementing change. This review did provide a valuable resource for people in the field and expanded their knowledge of what was available for them. It was, though, a lengthy and complex document for busy practitioners. But attempts were made to show how some approaches could be used through case studies in differing fields.

The vast majority of Change Management Models available for use in health care were not devised in the healthcare context. They tended to be from the business world and tended to focus on changing thinking and on specific outcomes rather than on people and how they respond to change. There are some health care specific models from the UK and across the globe. These similarly failed to consider that people are at the heart of change and some have complicated instructions with many layers of advice, the NHS model is such an example. We have shown that models are adaptable and can be used in a variety of settings, with different types of change and with different professions. However, many of these models have no consideration of the people who will need to engage both cognitively and emotionally with the change if it is to be successful. In many, the language used is robotic in tone, introduced hierarchically, instructing staff to follow particular steps, and there is little evidence of engagement with the wealth of experience, skill or knowledge of the workforce, who understand the culture and complexity of the situations they are working in.

There are Change Management Models in this genre that do consider both the cognitive and the emotional elements of change but the form in which these models are presented for use in practice do not necessarily provide the scope or opportunity for agents of change to focus on both people's thinking and feeling. For example, Kotter's model identifies that change cannot take place without addressing the head and the heart, and indeed he suggests that the heart is more significant in change management. However, his business model does not give emotions a place in his eight steps, so busy practitioners, change agents using the model, would not be aware of his views on the importance of emotions unless they have read his books. With Lewin's model, it is often presented simply as three stages to manage change without attention to group dynamics or action research.

While most models of change focus on cognitive engagement of staff, some do consider the wider person and include reference to how staff will respond emotionally to change. For example, there is a model focusing on the psychological cycle of emotion resulting from bereavement, in particular the grief cycle which is not linear but shows the emotional upheaval that can happen, seeing change as loss. This can be particularly useful to understand individual reactions to change. Others see change as a transition, for example Bridges model is based in the psychology of how people respond to change, but its rather narrow focus tends to make it unsuitable for complex changes in a large organisation. Appreciative Inquiry is another useful model, but its focus on the positive can deny the huge impact which change might be having on individuals, and that this impact will need to be addressed before change can be effective.

In health care, the language used for enacting change has tended to be fluid: modernisation, improvement, innovation, development, quality improvement and change. Whatever language is used, it is change that is required. In support of these different kinds of change, NHS Improvement has produced a host of tools and resources to support quality improvements. These tools have been cited as having a historic connection in the business world and could usefully apply to the NHS. There is enormous value for change agents and leaders to now have an extended range of improvement tools supported by a national body to aid change management. However, these are equally robotic in their approach and tone. They are directing people what to do without considering whether they are ready to enact service improvement, innovation or development. In effect, bringing about change without considering cognitive and emotional readiness for change.

The case for new thinking – cognitive and emotional readiness for change

In this book, we have considered how change management could potentially be successful. We believe this is an urgent matter and have argued for new thinking.

We believe the focus needs to be on people, that is human nature. That successful change management could potentially be achieved through cognitive and emotional readiness for change with the AC-W Change Management Model. This model enables assessment of cognitive and emotional readiness for change though a simple to use tool. Such knowledge will then help change leaders to understand the state or level of cognitive and emotional readiness of their workforce which means that they can put in place preparedness programmes, which then enables success in the implementation of change.

People bring about change, not tools, policies, strategies, approaches or models. But as we argued earlier, one gets the sense that the people in the NHS do not matter when it comes to change. They are unimportant, not valued, not consulted, with no sense that they can contribute useful input to proposed change, as if detached rationality should be the only and prevailing philosophy in managing change in healthcare. This is a negative way of approaching change. Firstly because it treats the workforce as machines, to obey whatever the leader directs, secondly, it ignores both the cognitive and emotional elements of change and often it ignores emotion entirely as something that might get in the way of implementing change. Emotional reactions to change are often interpreted as resistance to change, rather than as realistic assessments of the likely impact of change within the health care setting.

We believe that this is completely the wrong approach to take. Human nature operates with both heart and mind. Cognition and emotion operate in tandem, not separately. Thus, the AC-W Change Management Model encompasses both cognition and emotion. But, with emotion given so little attention, it is essential that we show its importance and relevance to our approach to change management. Change is emotional and impacts people in many ways and sometimes to a considerable extent. Evidence points to the fact that if managed well, emotions can enhance, improve and promote change management. With caring being the essence of the practitioner's role and contributing to high emotional labour, the emotional needs of practitioners need to be addressed if change is to be successful. Here we are considering normal human nature when changes are happening.

Nature of emotion

It is not surprising that emotion is a neglected feature in healthcare. Through exploring the nature of emotion, we found that historically emotion has not had a good press with ancient philosophers viewing it as controlling us instead of us within our control, something that impacts our judgements, pointless or as separate from the mind. Though perspectives have shifted, this is not often reflected in the underpinning philosophy in the array of change management approaches and how change is managed by leaders of change. One could further argue that the incessant policy changes thrown at us by politicians are treating us as machines rather than as humans with emotions.

Change and emotion

Change and emotion are interwoven. We examined the impact of change on people across a range of health care settings and groups, including managers. With high levels of change occurring in health care, we expected to find a huge amount of evidence on the benefits and drawbacks of health care changes. There was a paucity of literature about this for health care settings. However, we found ample evidence linking change to physical, mental and psychological effects in organisations. These were mainly negative with little, if any, evidence of positive outcomes. While the evidence in this arena was in the main on organisational changes, many of the outcomes will be familiar and will have been experienced by people within the health care setting. Within health care settings, and the NHS specifically, much of the evidence was during the 1990s and early 21st century. However, evidence has been slowly growing recently.

We further examined the evidence around emotion and change management. There was support for the idea that acknowledging and addressing emotions during change can lead to successful change management. Research in this arena suggests that the emotional intelligence of the leader, communication in an equally emotionally intelligent manner, the involvement and engagement of staff which can create an emotional connection with work, can all improve change management.

Caring is emotional and emotional labour is high and an essential aspect of health care roles. Caring is after all the essence of health practitioners' roles and what many specifically signed up for. While this can be both a rewarding and satisfying part of the work, it can be demanding and lead to physical and mental ill effects for the health care professional, especially when its importance is not acknowledged by those in more senior roles. We outlined the negative and positive impacts as evidenced in the literature. One of the major challenges for managers is that emotional labour cannot be 'measured' and so it is often disregarded, and yet forms a significant part of the practitioner's role. However, emotional labour does not just occur in relation to the health care worker's role in caring for patients, but also in their interactions with the multidisciplinary team and in facing demands from the organisation.

To reiterate we believe that human nature operates with both heart and mind. Cognition and emotion operate in tandem, not separately, which is the underpinning approach to the AC-W Change Management Model. People are complex beings, needing to understand the purposes of proposed changes, able to input ideas and rational arguments to improve such changes, but also likely to have personal and work-related emotional reactions to proposed changes within their working environment which will have impact on their everyday lives. Acknowledging the abilities of the workforce and their unique potential contributions and desire for change which impacts positively on patients, should enable leaders of change to work more collaboratively with staff. Effective management of change is to manage emotions, one's own and those of employees, not deny their existence.

Readiness is distinct from notions of resistance. The unique positions held by practitioners may well enable them to see that proposed changes will create challenges or have negative consequences unforeseen by leaders. If leaders are able to stop themselves expecting resistance, and instead identify where employees are expressing genuine concerns, not addressed by the proposed change, then the proposed changes can be adjusted with the wisdom of the workforce.

The notion of readiness encompasses beliefs, attitudes and intentions and while there is no consensus on the notions, the original view was that readiness was cognitive only with no role for emotion. Ideas of cognitive and emotional readiness are gaining ground. Writers who once believed readiness to be cognitive only have revised their view to include emotion. However, there is a huge shortfall in change models and research in the field on emotional readiness. Researchers and writers now agree that cognition and emotion are interwoven and interdependent and this relationship underpins the AC-W change model. Instead of leaders using their skills and resources to combat so-called resistance to change, these may be better used in creating cognitive and emotional readiness for change.

A new way of change – cognitive and emotional readiness

The AC-W Change Management Model is about cognitive and emotional readiness for change. Human nature is given centre stage in the model and this is surrounded by nine spokes which are the key principles underpinning organisations. This focus on human nature reminds change leaders that it is people who bring about change, and their thoughts and feelings in the change process are critical and must be considered. The model is intended to support the entirety of change. Thus, by initially assessing cognitive and emotional readiness for change with the accompanying tool, the change agent should be armed with data which will give an indication of the state of cognitive and emotional readiness which will then allow a programme of preparedness to be put in place to enable people to feel equipped to take the next step of implementing the change.

We wanted to demonstrate the model in action through the entirety of the change process, using case studies. However, we wanted to home in on the importance of the initial stage in change management, that is having the knowledge of cognitive and emotional readiness in their staff group, as this will determine the rest of the change process.

In the first change involving a redesigned medical unit, we gathered data about the thinking and feelings of practitioners, managers, senior managers and clinicians who actually experienced the change (retrospectively) to assess their cognitive and emotional readiness for that change. The second change was rather complex, involving the creation of a new foundation Trust, the relocation of children's community services and the CCG imposing a new service. Similarly, here we met with a range of staff and we collected data about peoples thinking and their feelings during a (real time) change in community and primary care. For the final change, we met with a child health and a mental health practitioner to see how practitioners could use the model to prepare clients for a lifestyle change. Thus, we used the tool to assess cognitive and emotional readiness of their clients (prospective).

These changes revealed the lack of emotional readiness for change amongst practitioners. There were common threads across all staff and all settings, irrespective of level of position held in the organisation, in community and primary care, acute or mental health settings which reflected the actual thinking and feelings of staff in the different settings. Overwhelmingly staff were experiencing or had experienced negative emotions about the change with no positive feelings reported. The range, intensity and outcomes were the same whether staff were in primary care and community or the acute sector. In the case of the retrospective change, these feelings were still present some months later after the medical division was redesigned.

However, the sources for this emotional unreadiness for change were different between the two settings. While in the acute sector it was due to loss of qualified colleagues, unqualified staff taking on previous nursing roles, ineffective general management, poor nursing leadership and the burden of emotional labour, in the primary care sector it was related to heavy workload, three major changes occurring simultaneously, invisibility of senior managers, loss of existing teams, regrading of posts, change of location of the team, increased workload, travelling longer, new responsibilities with the CCG without shedding any current responsibilities and loss of autonomy within their professional roles.

There was a lack of readiness of management and professional leadership at all levels and in these respective organisations to lead these changes. In these same changes, it showed the lack of readiness of the collective leadership to lead the change in the organisation, to involve staff, to empower them, to engage them, to support them, to address their responses to the change, some of which could have been anticipated. In essence their lack of readiness for effective change management. Leaders in the main focused on managing tasks, steps and outcomes rather than people.

There was lack of readiness of the tools regarding communication, and a lack of evidence of skills and knowledge of the importance of communication by leaders both in the acute sector and community and primary care. There was no communication with frontline employees, no attempt to engage staff, involve, empower or engage them with change. The engagement and involvement of the workforce by leaders of healthcare has the potential to result in a healthier and happier workforce and to enable more effective change, and thus to improve people's cognitive and emotional readiness for change.

The research exploring the use of the AC-W change management tool also found a poor culture of continuous readiness for change. In other words, despite the numerous changes which had been attempted, there was no sense that managers had prepared staff for ongoing change. Similarly, there was scant attention to embedding change. Change was a task to be ticked off, rather than a process which required ongoing effort over prolonged time to ensure change was sustained. The vast array of Change Management Models and literature available to help manage change were not used in managing change. Thus, despite the considerable effort and publications about change, it seems that they have not led to improvements in the way change is managed in health care settings.

Both the retrospective and real time case studies of change revealed failings in these organisations to prepare their employees for change.

While we showed the model in action through the entire change process and began by assessing cognitive and emotional readiness, to setting out the preparedness programme and implementation of the change. We were also keen to demonstrate that AC-W Change Management Model could be used in conjunction with other Change Management Models.

This began with a change in primary care, the change involved implementing an App to aid self-management of type 2 diabetic patients involving both primary care and the acute sector. We met with staff in primary and community care and the acute sector and used the AC-W Change Management Model to assess their readiness for change. Together with Lewin's three-stage change model, we set out the preparedness programme and implementation of that change. In the second change, we had already used the AC-W tool to assess cognitive and emotional readiness for change in the acute sector (redesign of a medical unit) and thus had the data of their readiness at hand. We therefore continued with the AC-W Change Management Model to show the preparation that was necessary and the implementation of that change, demonstrating that this model could be used for managing change from inception to completion. The third change involved implementing an innovative scheme to attract and retain staff in mental health, involving both the local mental health Trust and mental health services in primary care and community. We met with staff and used the AC-W Change Management Model to assess their cognitive and emotional readiness for change. With Kotter's eight stage change model, we set out the preparations needed and the implementation of that change.

For all of these three changes, there was lack of cognitive and emotional readiness for these changes. Staff emotions were in a negative state towards the change, the leadership was autocratic and focused on management rather than leading. Similarly, there was lack of engagement, involvement and empowerment, so staff were not ready for the change. What was striking was the similarity in lack of readiness for these three changes to the feedback from staff in the retrospective and real time change. The findings gathered from these changes concur with the evidence in the literature. Change at the whim of leaders, for short-term gain, and in a piecemeal fashion might create more disengagement and dissatisfaction amongst staff.

Summary and recommendations

With the evidence pointing to a lack of success in healthcare change, leaders of change need to explore new ways of managing change that focuses on people rather than using an autocratic style of management and change tools, techniques, approaches, models and theories that treat people as machines. Health care organisations need to have a change strategy in place. This needs to include an organisation wide plan with the scale, breadth and timing of changes connected. Any change plans need to be informed by an understanding of the workforce's emotional and cognitive readiness for change in all settings and at all levels in Trusts and organisations.

The AC-W Change Management Model offers change leaders the opportunity to manage change in a people-centred manner from inception to completion, through assessing the workforce's emotional and cognitive readiness for change. Through the simple to use tool for busy practitioners, data from staff sharing their thinking and feeling on readiness for change can aid change leaders in measuring the level of readiness for change which in turn can help determine an implementation that can potentially lead to successful change.

Using the simple to use tool could not only have a therapeutic benefit in releasing pent up feelings when change is enacted, giving a voice to the workforce but helping them feel engaged and involved in the change implementation plan.

The AC-W model can also be used in conjunction with other change approaches. Prior to any change, assessing the workforce's emotional and cognitive readiness for change through the simple to use tool for busy practitioners could provide valuable information of how the workforce are thinking and feeling, which can then help build the implementation plan.

The paucity of literature on the impact of healthcare changes needs addressing. It is surprising that with such a long history of healthcare change with little success that research has not focused on answering the simple question of why change success is so poor. Therefore, academics, writers, researchers and practitioners need to rise to the challenge in this arena. With the volume of change models, theories, approaches, tools and techniques available to manage change in the main from the business sector, more research is needed to assess the effectiveness of these in a health care context.

With few change approaches designed within the healthcare context, research is needed to measure the effectiveness of these within health care. In particular the NHS model, which seem complex and daunting for practitioners and the PDSA model seems procedural in its approach. Both not acknowledging the importance of people, their feeling and thoughts. The AC-W change model is a new approach to change management in health care which has not been tested on a large scale in Trusts and organisations. Thus, research on its implementation in change management needs to be evaluated in all settings and with individuals at all levels in Trusts and organisations.

Reference

Nuffield Trust, 2021. *Briefing: July 2021. Second Reading of the Health and Care Bill*. London: Nuffield Trust. Available at: www.nuffieldtrust.org.uk/files/2021-07/nuffield-trust-briefing-for-health-and-care-bill-second-reading.pdf

INDEX

Note: Page numbers in *italics* indicate a figure and page numbers in **bold** indicate a table on the corresponding page.

Accounts Commission recommendations 8–9
AC-W Change Management Model 92, 98–99, 109, 125, 179, 188–191; applications of 111, 129; for app to aid patients in primary care 155; culture of readiness for continuous change 120–122, **122**; development of 131; direction of change in frontline 122–123; emotional centre 98, 110–111, 125; engagement and involvement of people 118–119, **119**; as 'hub' and 'spokes' model *110*, 110–112; inter-organisational communication forums 119–120, **121**; leadership skill development 115–117; leadership styles 115–117, 157; management skill development 115–117; meeting organisation's business 123–124; need for 112–114; organisational values 118–119; prospective change case study 144–148; purpose of 98, 111, 125; real time change case study 133–135, **135**; for redesign of medical unit 160, 162, 169; retrospective change case study 131–133, **133**; structure and rationale 114–124; underpinning philosophy of 114, 131; valuing everyone equally 118–119, **119**; vision building 118–119, **119**
analysis-think change, flow of 111

Appreciative Inquiry 66, 69–70, 74
app to aid patients in primary care, case study of 152; assessment of readiness for change **155**, 155–156; communication forums 157; expertise development 157; implementation phase of 158; involvement, engagement and empowerment 157; meetings with staff 156–157; planning phase of 153–155; reinforcing change 158–159
Aristotle 78
autocratic leadership 116

behavioural theories of change management 66, 75; conditioning 70; Maslow's hierarchy of human needs 72–73; nudge theory 71–72; positive reinforcement, notion of 71; Rogers' work 73; self-efficacy, concept of 71; social learning theory 72; staged models of change 72
belief 94
'Best Practice Change Management Guidelines, The' 54
Big Three model of organisational change 51
Blair government reforms to NHS: achievements of 2; areas of 2; concerns with 2, 3; consumerism and competition 22–23; modernisation of NHS 179; shift towards primary care 34–35

Index **193**

Bridges Transition Model 68
British public, views of NHS 37–38
Burnes, Bernard 53

Canadian health care system, change management within 56
Canadian Health Service Research Foundation 56
Cannon-Bard 78
care, six Cs of 29
Care Quality Commission 7
CCGs (Clinical Commissioning Groups) 6, 9, 36, 137, 181, 183
change 16; barriers to 54; and emotion 187–188; failure rates for 42; impact on emotions 77; as loss 67; *see also* emergent approach to change; emotion; emotional and cognitive readiness for change
change leaders 2, 17, 38, 50, 53, 93, 95, 113, 115, 120, 123, 182, 186, 188; bottom-up approach 111; change management best practice for **117, 119, 121–124**; creating readiness for change 97–98; as effective communicators 120, 141; leadership styles 117, 125; people-centred approach to change 113–114
change management 92, 178; within Canadian health care system 56; complexity of 13; failure 181–186; lack of quality research for 51; managing emotions 85; people-centred approach to 113–114, 116
change management approaches 1, 42–43; emergent approach to 49–53; Kotter's model 46–48; Lewin's model 43–45; organisational development 48–49
change management tools: cognition 15–16; emotion 14
change models 15, 43–48
change readiness *see* readiness for change
CHSRF *see* Canadian Health Service Research Foundation
clan-type culture 23, 25
Clarke, Kenneth 34
classical conditioning 70
clients in community and primary care: attention to emotions 146–147; change model for 145; communication of 148; data collection for **144**, 144–145; empowerment of 147; holistic needs of 145; involvement and engagement of 147; leadership of 147
'clinical governance' 24
coalition government's record, NHS reform 32

cognition: cognitive elements 16–17, 77; cognitive engagement 93; and emotion, link between 73–74, 78–79
cognitive and emotional readiness for change *see* emotional and cognitive readiness for change
cognitive readiness for change 17, 43, 47, 54, 65, 74, 91, 94–95, 98–99
cognitive theories 66, 70
collaboration 7, 30
collaborative leadership 8
communication 96, 119–120; and collectivism 26–28; community and primary care 141–142; forums, inter-organisational 119–120, **121**; large acute hospital trust 141–142; in real time change 120; in retrospective change 120; *see also* open communication
community and primary care, organisational and practice change in 132; attention to embedding change 142; change management models for 143; communication 141–142; culture of readiness for continuous change 142; empowerment 140–141; engagement and involvement 140–141; lack of leadership 138–140; negative emotions 137–138; participants contributed to **135**; themes emerged for 136; valuing of individuals and teams 140–141; vision 140–141
community pharmacy, Kotter's model for practice change in 47
compassionate leadership 116–117
Competing Values Framework 23, 28
competition within NHS 7, 22–23, 34
conditioning, classical and operant 70
conflict and power 30
culture: issues impacting 22; negative impact of 22; of readiness for continuous change 120–122, **122**

'death of despair' phenomenon 10
democratic leadership style 116
Department of Health (DoH) 32
Descartes 78
devolution 8–9, 26–29, 184
diagram of AC-W Change Management Model *110*
digital health records 10
drug related deaths 10

electronic care plans, emotions related to 83
electronic rostering 54–55
emergent approach to change 49–53, 59–60, 91; Big Three model of

organisational change 51; from bottom of organisation 49–50; competitive advantage of 52; concept of receptivity 52, 53; evidence-based practice 53; global response to a pandemic 50; Pettigrew and Whipp's model 52; planned approach vs. 49, 50; strategic change 51–52; theoretical models 50–51; for unplanned event 50

emotion 92; in acute sector and community and primary care 136–138; addressing 79; and cognition, link between 17, 78–79, 112, 113–114; historical perspective of 77–78; in models of change 67; nature of 186–188; physical and psychological experiences of 78; role during change process 111; of workforce 16, 77; see also emotional and cognitive readiness for change; resistance to change

emotional and cognitive readiness for change 1–2, 14, 16–17, 47, 54, 65, 74, 91, 106, 114, 178, 185–186, 188–190; importance of assessment for 130–131; leaders' roles in creating 97; model for 17, 98–99, 109–124; personal change **104–105**, 130, 148–149; retrospective and real time change on 136–143; strategy of preparedness for 143–144, 148–149; tool for assessment of 99–100, **101–104**, 131

emotional elements of change 16–17, 48, 53, 61, 67, 77; action research 66; Appreciative Inquiry 69–70; Bridges Transition Model 68; grief cycle 67; link to cognition 73–74, 93, 113, 185

emotional engagement with change 55–56, 93

emotional impact of change 81–83

emotional intelligence 48, 112; definitions of 83–84; development of 81; of health care staff 84–85; of leaders 84; receptivity to change with 84

emotional labour 16, 77, 79–81; challenges of 80; concept of 79; impact on health of workers 80–81; of nurses 79–80

emotional readiness for change 43, 96

emotional responses to change 82

emotions associated with change 78

employees' contracts, NHS policy change impact on 11

employees' wellbeing, NHS policy change impact on 11

employers 16

engagement and involvement 118

England, life expectancy in 10

face to face communication 120
Fair to All policy 26
Francis Inquiry Report 6, 22, 23, 24

'garage' model 26
General Practice 35
general practitioners see GPs
general public and NHS 37–38
Goleman, Daniel 65, 78–79, 83
'Good Medical Practice' 29
GPs 9, 11–12, 33, 34, 36–37, 152, 183; as commissioner of services 33; at creation of NHS 32; workload, policy changes impact on 12
grief cycle 65, 67, 74
grieving process 81

HCPC see Health and Care Professions Council
Health and Care Bill 2021-2022 10
Health and Care Professions Council 27, 29
health and safety investigation branch 7
Health and Social Care Act of 2012 3, 36
Health and Social Care Bill 32
health behaviours: nudge theory and 66; staged models of change for 72; transtheoretical change model and 66
healthcare change and change models 53–57
health care contracts 23
Healthcare Environment Inspectorate 7
Healthcare Financial Management Association 8
Healthcare Improvement Scotland 7, 8
healthcare policies 32, 35, 57, 178, 181; impact on health care quality 9–10; impact on staff health and wellbeing 11–14, 32; over period 1983-1997 **3**; over period 1997-2009 **4–5**; see also NHS
health effects of change 78
health professions, values of 29
healthy choices, nudge theory supporting 71–72
healthy lifestyle as professional expectation 12
Heiddegar, Martin 78
HFMA see Healthcare Financial Management Association
hierarchical structures 25, 46–47, 55
hierarchy of human needs 72
Hume, David 78
Husler, Edmund 78

ICSs see integrated care systems
improvement process 55
integrated care systems 6–7
Integration Authorities 8

internal market 33–35
inter-organisational communication forums 119–120, **121**
interprofessional problem solving 30

James-Lang theory 78
job satisfaction 116; and emotional intelligence, link between 81; feedback of appreciation 79

Kotter's model of planned change 46–48, 51

Labour party 32
large acute hospital trust, organisational change in: attention to embedding change 142; change management models for 143; communication 141–142; culture of readiness for continuous change 142; empowerment 140–141; engagement and involvement 140–141; lack of leadership 138–139; negative emotions 136–138; participants contributed to 131, **133**; redesign of medical unit 132; themes emerged for 136; valuing of individuals and teams 140–141; vision 140–141
Large Scale Change, model for 55
Lazarus 74, 78
leadership 96, 125; best practice for 117; change management by 115; in community and primary care 138–140; development 115, 117; and emotional intelligence 84; in large acute hospital trust 138–139; medical doctors 69; in retrospective and real time change study 116; styles 115–117, 157
lean in health care, articles on 58
legislation since devolution in Scotland 8
Lewin, Kurt 43–45, 48, 66, 93
Lewin's model of change 43, 53, 65, 74; action research 66; criticism of 44, 66; resistance to change in 93; success of 45; three-stage process of 44–45
life expectancy: across UK countries 10; and healthy life expectancy, gap between wealthy and poor 10
London Procurement Programme 54

Maslow's hierarchy of human needs 72–73
medical unit, redesign of 152, 159–169; CEO role in 161; change implementation 169; plan development for 159; planning phase of 160; project director role in 161; project manager role in 162; readiness for change assessment for 162–168, **163**

mental health nurses, challenges for 30
mental health problems and organisational change, link between 82
mental health staff, scheme to attract and retain 152, 169; change process for 170; communicate for 'buy in' 174; empowerment action 175; guiding team building 172–173; readiness for change assessment **172**; regular interaction 175; sense of urgency for 171; short-term wins 175; vision for staff wellbeing 174; working groups for 173
Mid Staffordshire NHS Foundation Trust, Francis Inquiry Report into failings at 6, 22
midwives, values for high quality care 30

National Framework for Service Change in Scotland 26
National Health Service *see* NHS
National Institute for Health and Clinical Excellence 3, 54
nature of emotion 16, 77–79, 186
negative emotions 16, 67, 74, 79, 81, 83, 136–137, 136–138, 145–146; *see also* emotion
negative reinforcement of behaviour 70
NFSCS *see* National Framework for Service Change in Scotland
NHS 1, 91; challenges of 31; complexity of 21, 38; and general public 37–38; goals of establishing 31; government as administrator of 32; Management Board 33; money taken out of 23; re-organisation of 32–33; subjected to efficiency savings 66; under Thatcher government 33–34; universal health service of 33
NHS Change Model 53, 55
NHS Commissioning Board 36–37
NHS Constitution for England 25
NHS England 6, 53; Blair government reforms to 2; challenges experienced by 28; Change Model 54; 'church' model of 26; complexity of 21; concentration of power in 28; establishment of 36; Executive Summary for 53; 'garage' model of 26; policy changes 1; proposals for change within 6; top-down regulation, criticism of 8, 27; values of 26–27
NHS Executive 34, 36
NHS Five Year Forward View policy 36
NHS Foundation Trusts 3, 6, 11, 22, 36, 133
NHS Improving Quality group 55

196 Index

NHS Northern Ireland 9; challenges faced by 28; health policy reviews 28; values of 26, 28

NHS policy changes 38–39, 91; during 1948–1983 32–33; during 1983–1987 33; during 1987–1997 33–34; during 1997–2010 34–35; under coalition government 35–36; during COVID-19 pandemic 36–37; internal market 33–35; shift towards primary care 34–35; under Thatcher government 33–34

NHS Quality Improvement Scotland 59

NHS Scotland: challenges faced by 27; frontline staff involvement in 27; policy changes 7–8; small-scale implementation of change in 59; values of 25–27

NHS Trusts 3, 24, 33–34, 118, 132, 159

NHS Wales: challenges faced by 28; policy changes 8–9; values of 26–28

NICE *see* National Institute for Health and Clinical Excellence

Nietzsche, Fredrick 78

Nightingale hospital 37

NMC *see* Nursing and Midwifery Council

Northern Ireland: health policy, NHS 26, 28; life expectancy in 10; political structures of 28

nudge theory 71–72, 75

Nuffield Trust 10, 25, 27, 181

nurses 11, 24, 29; emotional experiences on organisational change 138; emotional labour of 79–80; healthy lifestyle as professional expectation 12–13; leadership of 12; and medical professionals, conflict between 30; recruitment crisis 12, 13; resilience promotion strategies 13; resistance to change 93

Nursing and Midwifery Council 27, 29

Nursing Workforce Standards 23

OD *see* organisational development

OECD: criticism of NHS England top-down regulation 8; on health care quality measurement 9

open communication 30

openness from leaders 93

organisational change 50, 81; health effects of 82; mental health problems with 82; *see also* large acute hospital trust, organisational change in

organisational culture: diversity of 24–25; elements of 22; and health care effectiveness, link between 24; Northern Ireland health care system 28; in Primary Care Trusts 25; sustainable change, guiding principles for making 25

organisational culture, change in 31, 38; complexity of 23; consumerism and competition 22–23; emotions experienced during 82–83; rational style culture 23; values, norms and assumptions 24

organisational development 15, 48–49

organisational readiness for change 15

organisational values 118–119

participative leadership 53

passions with primeval drives 78

patient-centred care 30

patient outcomes: and human resources practices, link between 11, 13; and staff satisfaction, Lean's role in 58

PCG *see* Primary Care Group

PCTs 25, 34–35, 36, 118, 133, 179–180

PDSA (plan, do, study, act) cycle of incremental change 55, 56, 58–60

perineal suturing technique, change to 59

planned approach to change 91; Kotter's model 46–48; Lewin's model 43–45; limitations of 49; organisational development 48–49

positional power, resistance to change for abuse of 93

positive culture 22

positive reinforcement of behaviour 65, 70

primary care 3, 152; drive to promote 56; emotion and 136–138; leadership in 138–140; quality improvement activities in 58; shift towards 34–35; *see also* app to aid patients in primary care, case study of; clients in community and primary care; community and primary care, organisational and practice change in

Primary Care Group 34, 179

Primary Care Trusts *see* PCTs

PRINCE2 54–55

professional groups 11, 16, 38; challenges for 30–31; codes and standards of conduct for 29; collaborative work 29–30; complexity of 21; diversity in culture between 24; impact of policy change on 12–13; values of 26–27, 29–30; view of NHS philosophy 24

professional silos 29

project management approach to change management 123

project management tool 54–55
prospective change 48, 92, 99, **104–105**, 111, 131, 151; *see also* clients in community and primary care
public dissatisfaction with NHS 37–38
public health 7, 36

QIS *see* Quality Improvement Scotland
Quality and Outcomes Framework of 2004 34
Quality Improvement Scotland 7
quality improvement tools and techniques 57–60; emergent approach to change 59–60; financial savings 57; lean methodology 57–58; PDSA model 58–59

readiness, notion of 91
readiness for change 16, 54, 56, 178; cognitive 95–96; cognitive perspective 96; concept of 16–17, 46; definition of 94; emotional responses to 96; failing to consider 59; at individual level 95; leaders' roles in creating 97–98; at organisational level 95–96; *vs.* resistance to change 93; theorising organisational 94–95; transtheoretical model of 72; *see also* emotional and cognitive readiness for change
real time change 115, 116, 118, 130; communication in 120; introduction of new scheme 169–176; tool for assessment of emotional and cognitive readiness of 99, **102–104**; *see also* community and primary care, organisational and practice change in
Regional Hospital Boards 32
resistance management 92
resistance to change: organisational change 120; *vs.* readiness for change 93; reasons of 92–93; by workforce 92–94; *see also* emotion
retrospective change 99, 118; communication in 120; redesign of medical unit 159–169; *see also* large acute hospital trust, organisational change in
Ross, Elizabeth Kübler 67

Scotland: drug related deaths in 10; health policy direction in 7–8; health policy, NHS 7, 8, 26–27, 59; life expectancy in 10
Scottish Patient Safety Programme 7

see-feel change, flow of 79, 111
self-management of type 2 diabetes *see* app to aid patients in primary care, case study of
senior managers, in English NHS hospital trusts 23
sensemaking 66, 73, 96, 99, 112
service development 1, 160, 165, 170
service improvement 1, 39, 132, 159, 164–165, 180, 185
service innovation 109, 111
Shared Delivery Plan, 2015–2020 9–10
shared leadership 116
SHAs *see* strategic health authorities
Singer-Schahter 78
situational leadership style 116
smoking ban, in public places 9
social care reforms 10
social conflict 48
social constructionism 69
social democracy 157
social enterprises, notion of 36
social learning theory 71, 72
staff experience and patient satisfaction, links between 11–12
staff health and wellbeing: and patient outcomes, link between 11–12; policy changes impact on 11–14, 32
staged models of change 72
statutory medical examiner system within NHS 7
strategic health authorities 36, 92–93
success factors for change 59
'support' staff 11
sustainable culture change, guiding principles for 25

teamwork and conflict 30
Timmins, Nicholas 32–34, 57
tool for assessing emotional and cognitive readiness for change 92, 99–100, **101–104**
top-down decisions about change 47
top-down style of management 13, 17, 21, 23, 46, 49
transformational leadership and emotional intelligence, link between 84
Transition Model 65, 68
transtheoretical model of behaviour change 72, 75
Triple Aim Framework 56–57
type 2 diabetes, self-management of *see* app to aid patients in primary care, case study of

UK Health policy changes: impact on health care quality 9–10; impact on staff health and wellbeing 11–14, 32; over period 1983-1997 **3**; over period 1997-2009 **4–5**

values associated with NHS 25, 31, 38; codes and standards of conduct 29–30; 'collaboration and collectivism' 26–27; 'communication and collectivism' 26–28; differences in 28–29; 'garage' model 26; of 'nothing about me, without me' 28
value statements 26
Virginia Mason Institute 58

Waldegrave, William 34
Wales: health policy, NHS 8, 26, 27–28; life expectancy in 10
workload and policy changes 12
World's Biggest Quango 32, 35

Printed in the United States
by Baker & Taylor Publisher Services